Recommendations for evidence-based endoscopic surgery

The updated EAES consensus development conferences

Springer

*Paris
Berlin
Heidelberg
New York
Barcelona
Hong Kong
London
Milan
Singapore
Tokyo*

Edmund Neugebauer, Stefan Sauerland (editors)
Hans Troidl (coordinator)

Recommendations for evidence-based endoscopic surgery

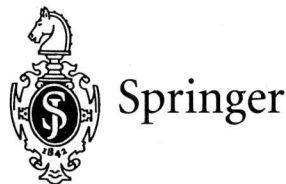 Springer

Edmund Neugebauer, Stefan Sauerland (editors)

Hans Troidl (coordinator)
11 Lehrstuhl für Chirurgie der Universität zu Köln
Biochemische und Experimentelle Abteilung
Ostmerheimer Straße 200, D 51109 Köln (Merheim)

Under the editing of Jean Mouiel & Alberto Montori

ISBN n° 2-287-59709-3 Springer-Verlag France, Berlin, heidelberg

© Springer-Verlag France, Paris, 2000
Printed in France

SPIN : 10772633
Cip requested

CONTENTS

Preface   1

Introduction . . . .
The Concept of the E.A.E.S. Consensus Development Conferences (CDC's)   3

Methodology   8
The E.A.E.S. consensus methods and their critical appraisal   8

Laparoscopic appendectomy   15
Consensus statements (1994)   17
Updating comments (2000)   19

Laparoscopic hernia repair   24
Consensus statements (1994)   26
Updating comments (2000)   28

Laparoscopic cholecystectomy   37
Consensus statements (1994)   39
Updating comments (2000)   41

**Laparoscopic antireflux surgery for gastroesophageal reflux disease
(GERD)**   47
Consensus statements (1996)   49
Updating comments (2000)   57

Diagnosis and treatment of common bile duct stones   63
Consensus statements (1997)   65
Updating comments (2000)   71

Diagnosis and treatment of diverticular disease   77
Consensus statements (1997)   79
Updating comments (2000)   85

Closing remarks and perspectives   90

PREFACE

PRESIDENTIAL ADDRESS

There is no doubt that the content of this EAES Consensus Development Conferences (CDC's) booklet represents an extremely important contribution to answering the following questions:

which area of endoscopic surgery requires quality assurance ?

what methodology should be employed ?

what further action is required ?

In order to try to answer these questions, the Executive Office of the EAES decided to appoint an "ad hoc" working group which started its activity in 1993.

Under the Presidency of Professor Hans Troidl and the scientific mandate of Professor Edmund Neugebauer the Consensus Development Conferences appeared as one of the essential educational programmes of the EAES. These were organized thanks to the scientific and secretarial assistance of the 2nd Department of Surgery, University of Cologne. Besides the appointed chairperson, each Conference was led by a clinical chairman who included surgical experts from various countries of Europe: J. Périssat, W. Wayand, A. Fingerhut, A. Paul, E. Eypasch, C.K. Kum.

Of course the EAES Congress Presidents and the panel members should be acknowledged for their important input in the Consensus Conferences.

From 1994 to 1998 six themes of endoscopic surgery have been assessed and their recommendation were presented and discussed during the European Congresses held in Madrid, Trondheim, Istanbul and in the World Congress Rome 98.

The themes were laparoscopic cholecystectomy, appendectomy, hernia repair, gastroesophageal reflux disease, common bile duct stones, diverticular diseases of the colon. The contents of these Conferences were published in Surgical Endoscopy, our official Journal.

In Linz 1999 an updating and a critical appraisal of consensus methods were included in the scientific program with a session devoted to: "Impact - What influence had the EAES CDC's?" and the contents were discussed with the audience by E. Neugebauer, S. Sauerland, B. Millat and H. Sitter.

The EAES Permanent Scientific Programme Committee has already decided to include during the European Congress Nice 2000 a preliminary report of experts' opinion conference on colonic cancer by elective laparoscopy and during the Postgraduate Course the experts' opinion on morbid obesity by laparoscopy. These two topics can represent also the basic point to organize in the near future two more EAES CDC's.

After the critical appraisal in Linz we should ask ourselves the same questions which were discussed during the scientific session: What influence had the EAES CDC's ? Why do we need CDC's at all ? How can we measure the impact of CDC's, What impact had the EAES CDC's on surgeons' performance and patients outcome? How to improve things !

Among the various educational activities of the EAES, the CDC's play a very important role and it is our opinion that the results of this work will be helpful in defining the most appropriate use of endoscopic surgery.

We would like to congratulate all the people involved in realizing such a great project which will be a "milestone" for surgeons.

This booklet certainly will represent the scientific basic rules ensuring a new successful era for the EAES CDC's. We are optimistic that this will come to pass and everyone will benefit from the results achieved.

On behalf of the EAES Executive and Administrative Boards we would like to express our deepest gratitude to the Cologne Group and to the Panel Members for their outstanding work.

JEAN MOUIEL, MD, FACS   ALBERTO MONTORI, MD, FACS
EAES Past President   EAES President

Introduction:

The Concept of the E.A.E.S.
Consensus Development Conferences (CDC's)

Authors:

E. NEUGEBAUER, Biochemical and Experimental Division, 2nd Department of
Surgery, University of Cologne (Germany)

Endoscopic surgery is often called a world-wide revolution or a break-through in surgical technique with significant positive effects on the outcome of surgical patients. There is nearly no field in surgery, which has not been approached by minimally-invasive techniques. However, it is one thing to show that a technique is feasible and safe, another to demonstrate that its application is of real benefit to the patient. Any new method has to be superior or at least equal to the conventional technique [1]. Early experiences of pioneers with this new tool has shown serious limitations and dangers of endoscopic surgical procedures, especially in less experienced hands [2]. Moreover, the advent of endoscopic surgery was accused to contribute significantly to the rising health care expenditure in times of short money. A comprehensive and critical assessment of a new methodology followed by guidelines on the best practice in the different fields on the current state of knowledge is therefore mandatory. For this reason already in 1993 the Executive Committee of the European Association for Endoscopic Surgery (E.A.E.S.), on the initiative of its former president H. Troidl, decided to critically assess systematically the progress of endoscopic surgery in the different developing fields of surgery. (This was an exception to the rule, as most professional societies avoid the issue of systematic evaluation of new technologies, because they fear to enter this minefield of medical, political, financial, and juridical consequences. [3]) The format chosen, for reasons given below, was the Consensus Development Conference (CDC).

Formal consensus methods are used by medical professional societies, private and third-party payers, biomedical research agencies, and others to assess state-of-the-art medical and surgical procedures and other technologies, to define standards and accepted medical practices, to bridge gaps and resolve disparities among research findings, and to establish coverage and reimbursement policies [4]. Their main common purpose is to define levels of agreement and disagreement on controversial subjects [5].

At least three consensus methods can be differentiated: the Delphi process developed by the Rand Cooperation [6; 7] and the Nominal Group Technique (NGT) [8] and Consensus Development Conferences (CDCs). The Delphi technique is an interactive survey process that uses controlled feedback to isolated, anonymous (to each other) participants. It does not provide the opportunity for classification of ideas and other benefits of face-to-face interactions. NGT requires bringing participants together. The product of NGT is a list of ideas and statements rank-ordered according to importance.

A method designed specifically to develop documents for use by health practitioners and policy makers is the Consensus Development Conference. The National Institutes of Health (NIH) had already started in 1977 a Consensus Development Program under the responsibility of the Office for Medical Applications of Research (OMAR) [9]. They had conducted 84 conferences already by the end of 1991 to integrate opinions of recognized experts in many controversial areas. Several countries in Europe (The Netherlands, Sweden, Denmark, UK, Finland, and Germany) followed the NIH model later on and remodeled the NIH methodology to adapt the technological assessment to the particular national context of the program. The method includes participation of speakers who present evidence, an audience that has the opportunity to comment on the evidence, and a panel that deliberates and produces a written statement based on its judgment. The methods of conference organization and conduct have evolved over the time. In general, however, each conference took 12-15 months to be organized and 2 1/2 days for the conference itself.

Although the idea of consensus development is common to all programs, the consensus development process and dissemination mechanisms differ across countries. Moreover, several attempts were made for strengthening consensus development in order to assess health technologies in a most unbiased way [10].

The processes by which consensus conferences are conducted can strongly affect the value and validity of the final product. Supporters of consensus argue that, when properly employed, consensus strategies can create structured environments in which experts are given the best available information, allowing their solutions to problems to be more justifiable and credible than otherwise [5]. However, major concerns are also obvious, and critics argue that the weaknesses outweigh the strength. Biases can be introduced at all levels of a consensus development process: (1) selection biases, particularly with respect to the choice of questions and panelists, (2) the examination of clinical or health services literature in order to construct a synthesis of what is known from published sources about the use of a technology - if a synthesis is done, it rarely relies upon formal meta-analysis or any quantitative process of combining evidence, (3) the process itself - the organization of the panels, the choice of leaders, the environment, and timing etc.

Depending on the criteria for making decisions, definition of consensus, formal voting or polling of panel members, the handling of disagreements, consensus statements very often represent the "lowest common denominator" of opinion. These points are often so mild and far from the cutting edge of progress and so well established that surely everybody must already know them. They provide little guidance as to exactly what ought to be done or as to exactly what their implications are. It must therefore be the goal of every consensus method to end up with consensus statements as specific as possible, i.e. exact information as to what something means, what should be done, and/or what data are required [11]. If no consensus is possible on certain points, the reasons must be stated.

Although the model of the NIH has been used extensively in other countries, it was also stated [12] that it has never been shown to produce replicable results or to be preferable to other models. Furthermore, it is time consuming and expensive. As with all approaches, there is always the potential for improvement of the process, particularly to enhance the inputs to the process and the methods by which issues and experts are identified in order to improve the final product. Formalizing the process by which consensus conferences are conducted not only enhances the credibility of the statements but also makes the process more scientifically defensible and replicable. Independent of the consensus method used, at least four essential elements must be covered to produce useful and credible outcomes [5]. There is a need to (1) carefully select problems that are amenable to solution by consensus; (2) closely monitor the choice of panels and their leaders; (3) identify justifiable consensus levels; and (4) make sure the findings are useful and accessible. The Executive Committee of the European Association for Endoscopic Surgery (E.A.E.S.) has decided to hold consensus development conferences with the premise to fulfill these demands. Up to now, six CDCs were performed since 1994 always in conjunction with its annual meetings. The methodology and the results are presented in this booklet of the E.A.E.S.

The methodology differs from the typical NIH format but instead combines elements from the nominal group technique, the Delphi process, and the NIH consensus development conferences program. One reason to change the format of the NIH program was that it is a time-consuming and expensive procedure. Moreover the field of endoscopic surgery is rapidly evolving. The E.A.E.S. felt that it ought to provide specific guidelines as soon as possible, which means early in the development of a new indication, where the evidence is sparse [13]. Serious considerations of the pros and cons of the different consensus methods described and our personal experience with the organization and conduct of consensus conferences [14; 15] forced us to develop a new, more practicable alternative. All essential elements of CDCs as mentioned above are covered: (1) topics were selected because of prevalence and socioeconomic impact, multidisciplinary interests, controversies in scientific aspects and "sufficient" research data; (2) panelists were chosen by the Educational/Scientific Committee of the E.A.E.S. by specific criteria; (3) consensus statements were developed in a structured way with provisional statements before the consensus meeting based on published literature; the consensus level was formulated on majority agreement of the panel when full agreement could not be obtained in the panel session; and (4) statements were formulated to be as specific as possible to provide useful guidelines.

Our experience with this new type of consensus development has shown that this format is indeed a more practicable alternative in comparison to other programs. The results achieved in these conferences are presented in this booklet together with updated versions in the year 2000 by the responsible chairpersons of the different conferences, based on a critical appraisal session at the annual conference of the E.A.E.S. in Linz/Austria, 1999.

References

1. Neugebauer E, Troidl H, Spangenberger W, et al. (1991) Conventional versus laparoscopic cholecystectomy and the randomized controlled trial. Br J Surg 78: 150-154.
2. Troidl H (1999) Disasters of endoscopic surgery and how to avoid them: error analysis. World J Surg 23: 846-855.
3. McKneally MF, McPeek B, Mulder DS, Spitzer WO, Troidl H, Organizing meetings, panels, seminars, and consensus conferences. In: Troidl H, McKneally MF, Mulder DS, et al. (Eds.),

Surgical research. Basic principles and clinical practice. 3rd Edition, Springer, Berlin, 1998, pp. 341-355.

4.   Committee of the Institute of Medicine - Council on Health Care Technology, Consensus development at the NIH: Improving the program, National Academy Press, Washington/DC, 1990, pp. 1-81

5.   Fink A, Kosecoff J, Chassin M, Brook RH (1984) Consensus methods: characteristics and guidelines for use. Am J Public Health 74: 979-983.

6.   Dalkey NC, The Delphi method: an experimental study of group opinion., Rand Cooperation, Santa Monica/CA, 1969

7.   Olsen SA, Group planning and problem solving methods in engineering management, J. Wiley & Sons, New York/NY, 1982

8.   Belbecq AG, Van de Veen AH, Gustafson DH, Group techniques for program planning, Scott Foresman, Glenview/IL, 1975

9.   Perry S, Kalberer JT, Jr. (1980) The NIH consensus-development program and the assessment of health-care technologies: the first two years. N Engl J Med 303: 169-172.

10. Goodman C, Barak SR, Improving consensus development for health technology assessment: an international perspective., National Academy Press, Washington/DC, 1990

11. Wortman PM, Vinokur A, Sechrest L (1988) Do consensus conferences work? A process evaluation of the NIH Consensus Development Program. J Health Polit Policy Law 13: 469-498.

12. McGlynn EA, Kosecoff J, Brook RH (1990) Format and conduct of consensus development conferences. Multi-nation comparison. Int J Technol Assess Health Care 6: 450-469.

13. Wortman PM, Smyth JM, Langenbrunner JC, Yeaton WH (1998) Consensus among experts and research synthesis. A comparison of methods. Int J Technol Assess Health Care 14: 109-122.

14. Neugebauer E, Troidl H (1989) Meran consensus conference on pain after surgery and trauma. A consensus conference with various clinical disciplines and basic research, 10-14 May 1988 in Meran, South Tyrol, Italy. Theor Surg 3: 220-224.

15. Neugebauer E, Troidl H, Wood-Dauphinee S, Eypasch E, Bullinger M (1991) Quality-of-life assessment in surgery: results of the Meran consensus development conference. Theor Surg 6: 123-137.

Methodology:

The E.A.E.S. consensus methods and their critical appraisal

Authors:

S. SAUERLAND, Biochemical and Experimental Division, 2nd Department of Surgery, University of Cologne (Germany);
E. NEUGEBAUER, Biochemical and Experimental Division, 2nd Department of Surgery, University of Cologne (Germany);

Consensus methods

E.A.E.S. consensus methods (1994-1998)

All CDCs that are summarized in this book have been conducted by the use of the same methodology. The whole process consisted of 9 steps, which were taken within a time-frame of about one year:

1. By majority voting, the E.A.E.S. scientific committee defined areas of endoscopic surgery, where the development of new technologies had led to uncertainty among surgeons, adn where a need for a focused opinion was perceived. Initially, the aim of the CDCs was mainly to prevent the ‚bush-fire'-like spread of new technologies, for which effectiveness was unproven and were the society feared potential harms related to the treatment.

2. The Cologne group (headed by E. Neugebauer and H. Troidl) then started to organise the consensus conference, by inviting a dozen or more field experts to participate. The criteria for selection were clinical expertise, scientific reputation and activity, community influence, and geographic location. While the first three panels were all-surgical, the following CDCs included also specialists from other disciplines.

3. When the panel had been selected, each expert was asked to describe his or her view about various aspects of the disease and treatment. We used a list of questions to structure this process. Experts were asked to search the literature and to cite relevant articles to support their arguments with valid data. They also were requested to rate the scientific strength of all studies cited. We defined different levels of evidence (**Table 1**). Different stages of a new technique were classified according to the stages of technology assessment: Feasibility (Is the procedure practically feasible?), efficacy (Does it provide benefit to patients at least in centres of excellence?), effectiveness (Is it beneficial in general practice?), and efficiency (Does it save money?)

4. From all the panelists' answers we compiled a preliminary statement, that was sent out to all panel members again. The panel members were unknown to each other to avoid interactions at this stage of process. This preliminary statement summarized the various opinions, included a list of references, a table of the according evidence levels, and a table with the technology assessment stages. Controversial issues were especially highlighted, but without giving the names of those experts, who disagreed with the rest of the panel.

5. Right before the annual E.A.E.S. conference began, the panel met for the first time personally. Under the guidance of a chairman and a moderator, who mainly blocked unduly long discussions, the experts discussed all aspects surrounding the CDC theme. The preliminary statements were reformulated until all experts agreed to them. Questions were no consensus was achievable, were defined as such.

Table 1: Rating scheme for published literature on therapeutic interventions

Strength of evidence (#A)	Strength of evidence (#B)	Study type
III	I	· Randomized controlled clinical trials (with power and relevant clinical endpoints)
II	II	· Non-randomized controlled clinical trial (either parallel or historical controls) · Case-control-studies
I	III	· Cohort studies with literature controls · Database analyses
	V	· Reports of expert committees
0	IV	· Case series / Case reports
	V	· Belief

Many different rating schemes have been proposed in the literature. The E.A.E.S. initially used the III-to-0-scheme (column #A, also known as AHCPR-scheme). Today, however, most schemes use level I to describe the highest level of evidence (column #B). They also have down-graded statements from experts or expert committees.

Often, this non-public group discussion lasted for many hours. The preliminary statement was rewritten during the night by a secretary of the organisers.

6. On the following day, the results of the panel discussion (the "pre-consensus statement") was presented to the public audience at the conference. The aim of this session was to familiarize surgeons with the newly developed recommendations and also to incorporate outlying opinions and objections, which sometimes were raised by individuals in the audience.

7. All new arguments, that had been brought up, were then non-publicly discussed by the panel and subsequently introduced into the recommendation. After this closing discussion the panel parted.

8. During the following months, the consensus statements were typed. The manuscript was then mailed to all panelists for final approval. Some CDCs were followed by a Delphi process, if important issues had not been addressed within the panel discussion or if formulations of certain parts of the text needed furhter refinement. (Within a Delphi process, a text is repeatedly send out to all experts for comment, and after each "round" the statement is reformulated until a convergence of opinion is visible.)

9. The final consensus statements were published in the official journal of the E.A.E.S., "Surgical Endoscopy". No other attempts were made to enhance CDC awareness and guideline use among European surgeons.

Methods for updating the consensus recommendations (2000)

There is a undeniable necessity to keep CDC statements up-to-date with the medical knowledge, which advances quickly, especially in the field of endoscopic surgery. However, as it was impossible for the original panels to meet again, it was decided that each chairman should compile updating comments on his theme. We suggested that these comments should be written on the basis of a thorough search of the available evidence. Some chairmen followed this suggestion, while other modified this approach. Details are described in the chapters itself.

Critical appraisal of consensus methods (1999)

European postal survey

Prior to the E.A.E.S. conference in Linz 1999, where a critical appraisal session was organised, the E.A.E.S. secretariat sent out a one-page questionnaire to all E.A.E.S. members. This questionnaire contained various questions about previous consensus statements, future directions, and general comments.

Only 309 of the 2200 questionnaires (14.0%) were returned to Cologne, mainly from University hospitals (57%). Two thirds of the respondents knew that the E.A.E.S. published the CDCs in "Surgical Endoscopy". Most surgeons remembered the themes of the past CDCs very well, although this varied: cholecystectomy (66%), gastro-esophageal reflux disease (53%), appendectomy (43%), hernia repair (41%), and common bile duct stones (32%). The fact that between 15 and 20% remembered E.A.E.S. CDCs on adhesiolysis, abdominal trauma, splenectomy, thoracoscopy, and colonic carcinoma (which have never taken place!), shows that surgeons don't put much emphasis on the agency that issues a CDC or guideline. Issues to be addressed by future CDCs were distributed equally among all above-mentioned themes, with one exception: In over half of the replies it was stated that laparoscopic surgery for colonic carcinoma should be assessed by a consensus panel.

Most E.A.E.S. members regard the CDC statements as clinical practice guidelines (82%), other found it important that the CDCs defined the current "state of the art" (55%) and also areas of uncertainty (48%). Others saw the CDCs as a means of surgical education for trainees (28%). Figure 1 shows that most E.A.E.S. members retrieve information from various sources.

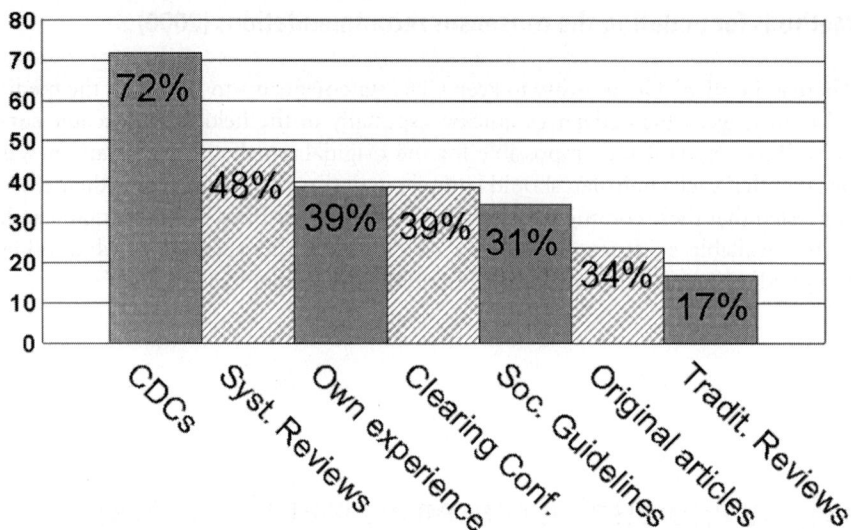

Figure 1: Answers to the question "What sources of evidence do you prefer for clinical decision-making?" Percentages add up to over 100%, as more than one answer was allowed. Some respondents added comments that they would use congress reports and informal exchange with colleagues for decions-making, too.

The vast majority of surgeons in this survey said that the CDC recommendations would help surgical education (90%), advance scientific progress (81%), and improve clinical practice (90%). However, only 67% admitted that the CDC statements did have an impact on their own clinical practice.

When asked to name the main disadvantages of the CDCs, about 20 replies commented on the ways by which the expert panels had been selected:

- "The experts are appointed on political grounds."
- "Experts' are nominated by other ,experts."
- "....some clique of people..."
- "Usually the outcome is dominated by one group."
- "Lack of interdisciplinary cross review."
- "Selection of experts determines results."

The results of this survey point out various weaknesses of the previous E.A.E.S. CDCs. The low response rate indicates that the survey results are still too optimistic due to response bias and also other forms of bias [1].

Incorporation of research evidence

Recent research indicated that "all areas of guideline development need improvement, greatest improvement is needed in the identification, evaluation, and synthesis of the scientific evidence" [2; 3].

By using the example of one E.A.E.S. consensus conference, we therefore investigated the retrieval rates for individual panel members [4]. After having compiled a complete list of relevant randomised controlled clinical trials (RCTs), we checked how many of these RCTs were identified by each of the panel members and correctly classified as level-I evidence. Of all those 49 papers that the experts believed to be RCTs, only 23 actually were RCTs. The sensitivity resp. specifity for correctly identifying an RCT was 0.21 (95%-CI: 0.11 to 0.30) resp. 0.80 (95%-CI: 0.64 to 0.95). RCTs that included the word "randomised" in their title were significantly more likely to be identified (relative risk: 1.31; 95%-CI 1.18 to 1.45).

Clarity of language

Clinicians can use clinical practice guidelines only, if these provide clearly formulated answers to clearly defined questions. We therefore assessed the unambigituity of the E.A.E.S. recommendations, although the definition of "unambiguity" itself is subjective.

Most statements were formulated according to the knowledge that supported the particular sentence. Panelists used various terms to vaguely describe the fact, that a recommendation was not without doubt: "in general", "under normal circumstances", "routine cases", "should", or "most cases". Today, many guidelines explicitly classify each statement according to the supporting evidence (e.g. "grade A recommendation"); this guideline transparency, however, was not given here.

The management of common bile duct stones (CBDS), which was discussed in 1994 (in connection with laparoscopic cholecystectomy) and again in 1997, provided the opportunity to compare these two recommendations for their content. We noticed one statement, which differed between 1994 and 1997: In 1994, the panel stated, that a history of pancreatitis is associated with a higher prevalence of CBDS. In 1997, a second panel said, that no evidence for this association exists.

Conclusions

We have critically assessed the E.A.E.S. consensus methods by various methods of investigation and from different points of view. Although methods have continually improved and are in some respect adequate or even good, the following points still have to be recognized as the main shortcomings in the consensus process in general:

1. Panel selection [5; 6]

2. Literature search [7; 8]

3. Transparency of recommendations [9; 10]

Improvements of our methodology are therefore necessary [11], and will be outlined in the final chapter of this booklet.

References

1. Adams AS, Soumerai SB, Lomas J, Ross-Degnan D (1999) Evidence of self-report bias in assessing adherence to guidelines. Int J Qual Health Care 11: 187-192.
2. Shaneyfelt TM, Mayo-Smith MF, Rothwangl J (1999) Are guidelines following guidelines? The methodological quality of clinical practice guidelines in the peer-reviewed medical literature. JAMA 281: 1900-1905.
3. Grilli R, Magrini N, Penna A, Mura G, Liberati A (2000) Practice guidelines developed by specialty societies: the need for a critical appraisal. Lancet 355: 103-106.
4. Sauerland S, Neugebauer E (2000) Consensus conferences must include a systematic search and categorization of the evidence. Surg Endosc (in press)
5. Fraser GM, Pilpel D, Kosecoff J, Brook RH (1994) Effect of panel composition on appropriateness ratings. Int J Qual Health Care 6: 251-255.
6. Leape LL, Park RE, Kahan JP, Brook RH (1992) Group judgments of appropriateness: the effect of panel composition. Qual Assur Health Care 4: 151-159.
7. Lomas J, Anderson G, Enkin M, et al. (1988) The role of evidence in the consensus process. Results from a Canadian consensus exercise. JAMA 259: 3001-3005.
8. Neugebauer EAM, Lefering R, McPeek B, Wood-Dauphinée S, Systematically reviewing previous work. In: Troidl H, McKneally MF, Mulder DS, et al. (Eds.), Surgical research. Basic principles and clinical practice. 3rd Edition, Springer, Berlin, 1998, pp. 341-355.
9. Grimshaw JM, Russell IT (1994) Achieving health gain through clinical guidelines. II: Ensuring guidelines change medical practice. Qual Health Care 3: 45-52.
10. Grimshaw JM, Russell IT (1993) Achieving health gain through clinical guidelines. I: Developing scientifically valid guidelines. Qual Health Care 2: 243-248.
11. Murphy MK, Black NA, Lamping DL, et al. (1998) Consensus development methods, and their use in clinical guideline development. Health Technol Assessment 2: i-iv, 1-88.

Laparoscopic appendectomy:

E.A.E.S. Consensus Development Conference (1997)[1,2] with updating comments (2000)

Conference organizers (1994):

E. Eypasch, Surgical Clinic Merheim, 2nd Department of Surgery, University of Cologne (Germany);

C. K. Kum, Department of Surgery, National University Hospital, Singapore (Singapore);

E. Neugebauer, Biochemical and Experimental Division, 2nd Department of Surgery, University of Cologne (Germany);

H. Troidl, Surgical Clinic Merheim, 2nd Department of Surgery, University of Cologne (Germany);

M. Miserez, Surgical Clinic Merheim, 2nd Department of Surgery, University of Cologne (Germany);

A. Paul, Surgical Clinic Merheim, 2nd Department of Surgery, University of Cologne (Germany);

Expert Panel (1994):

O.J. McAnena, Surgical Unit, University College Hospital, Galway (Ireland);

M. McMahon, Leeds Institute for Minimally Invasive Therapy, The General Infirmary, Leeds (Great Britain);

S. Attwood, Meath Hospital, Dublin (Ireland);

E. Schippers, Department of Surgery, Clinic RWTH, Aachen (Germany);

J. Jakimowicz, Department of Surgery, Catharina Hospital, Eindhoven (The Netherlands);

W. van Erp, Department of Surgery, Diaconessenhuis, Eindhoven (The Netherlands);

1) Held at the 2nd International Congress of the European Association for Endoscopic Surgery (E.A.E.S.), Madrid, Spain, 15-17 September, 1994

2) The original conference is published in Surg Endosc (1995) 9: 550-563.

P. Testas, Service de Chirurgie Generale, Centre Hospitalier Bicêtre, Le Kremlin-Bicêtre Cedex (France);
J. A. Lujan Mompean, Department of General Surgery, University Hospital "Virgen de la Arrixaca", El Palmar, Murcia (Spain);
J. S. Valla, Hôpital pour Enfants, Nice (France);

Updating comments (2000):

C. K. Kum, Department of Surgery, National University Hospital, Singapore (Singapore)

Consensus statements (1994)

Question 1: What stage of technological development is laparoscopic appendectomy (LA) at (in Sept. 1994)?

LA is presently at the efficacy stage of development, because most of the data on feasibility and safety originate from centers with a special interest in endoscopic surgery. More data on its use in general and district hospitals are needed to ascertain its effectiveness. Detailed analysis on its cost-effectiveness and cost benefits is also lacking. Although a very promising procedure, it is not yet the gold standard for acute appendicitis.

Question 2: Is LA safe and feasible?

1. There is no evidence in published literature that LA is any less safe than open appendectomy (OA).
2. Operation time, depending on the experience of the surgeon, is similar or longer than the open procedure.
3. Postoperative complications-e.g., bleeding, intraabdominal abscess, reoperation- are not more frequent than OA in the published literature. However, the morbidity associated with widespread application is not yet known.
4. LA is not contraindicated for perforated appendicitis. However, more data for this subgroup of patients is needed.
5. LA may be attempted for an appendiceal abscess by an experienced surgeon if the abscess is to be treated early. Conversion to open surgery should be undertaken when difficulties are encountered. Alternatively, delayed elective LA can be performed after resolution of the abscess with antibiotic therapy.
6. LA can be used in children. It should be performed only by surgeons with ample experience in adult LA. Smaller instruments should be available to improve safety and ergonomy.
7. The safety of LA during pregnancy is not established.
8. The indication for elective LA is the same as for open elective appendectomy.

Question 3: Is it beneficial to the patients?

1. Laparoscopy improves the diagnostic accuracy of acute right iliac fossa pain, especially in children and young women.
2. LA reduces the wound infection rate.
3. There is less postoperative pain in adults. There are no data in children.

4. Hospital stay is similar or less than OA.

5. LA allows earlier return to normal activities.

6. The laparoscopic approach may lead to less postoperative adhesions.

7. Cosmesis may be better than OA.

8. All in all, LA has advantages over OA. However, the potential for serious injuries must be appreciated and avoided in order to make the postoperative advantages worthwhile.

Question 4. What are the special technical aspects to be considered during LA?

The statements here are meant to be guidelines. The surgeon at the operating table has to be the ultimate judge as to what is safe to do.

1. Convert to open surgery if the appendix cannot be found.

2. At diagnostic laparoscopy, there is no obligation to remove the appendix.

3. Bipolar coagulation is a preferred mode of coagulating the artery. Monopolar diathermy may be safe if the appropriate precautions are taken. Use of clips alone or in combination with coagulation is the alternative. Suture ligation of the artery is usually unnecessary. Lasers and staples are not cost-effective.

4. When the base of the appendix is healthy and uninflamed, one properly applied preformed ligature is probably enough. If in doubt, use two loops. Metal clips alone are not recommended; staples are too expensive and not required in most cases.

5. The appendix should be transected at about 5 mm from the last preformed ligature. It is unnecessary to bury the stump.

6. To avoid wound infection, the appendix should be removed through the port or if too big, within a pouch.

7. Peritoneal toilet is recommended in cases of intraabdominal contamination.

8. The antibiotic policy should be the same as for open appendectomy.

Question 5. What are the training recommendations for LA?

1. LA should be part of the resident's curriculum.

2. At least 20 cases of LA are needed for accreditation in general surgery.

Summary

Laparoscopic appendectomy is an efficacious new technology. Its safety and feasibility have been shown in the published literature, mainly from centers with a special interest in endoscopic surgery. However, a few cases of serious complications have been reported. Surgeons should be aware of the potential dangers.

Benefits for the patients, especially in terms of more accurate diagnosis, reduction of wound infection, and earlier return to work, have also been shown in controlled trials, albeit with small numbers of patients. Its effectiveness, compared to open appendectomy, when applied generally to all grades of hospitals, remains to be seen. The cost-effectiveness of LA is not known. Although promising, it is not yet the gold standard for acute appendicitis.

Updating comments (2000)

Introduction

Laparoscopic appendectomy (LA) is nowadays the best studied laparoscopic procedure; perhaps even the most scrutinised surgical procedure ever. In 1994, there were already 6 randomised controlled trials (RCT) [1-6] and 13 prospective studies. To date, there are 38 RCTs involving more than 3300 patients. Most of these trial have been reported as full articles [1-25], while others are accessible only as abstracts, conference proceedings or theses [26-38].

The significant size of the literature on LA with differing results makes publication bias unlikely. More importantly, there are now 5 meta-analyses that are considered to represent the highest level of evidence-based medicine. [39-43]

Stage of Technological Development

Certainly, LA has reached the effectiveness stage. Of the 38 RCTs, 33 were published in English, 4 in German and 1 in French. In addition, there are numerous prospective and retrospective studies that have been published since 1990. Thus it was not only studied in a few specialised centres, but in various hospitals in different countries. Today, it is a common practice to perform a diagnostic laparoscopy for right iliac fossa pain, followed by laparoscopic appendectomy if the appendix is inflamed; and often even when the appendix appears normal. The main obstacle appears to be availability of equipment.

Safety and Feasibility

There are no significant changes from the statements of 1994. Safety and feasibility should have been improved with better equipment and more experience amongst surgeons. LA has been confirmed to be as safe as open appendectomy (OA).

Operation time is on the average 15-20 min longer than the open procedure. Postoperative complications are not more than OA. One of the authors was concerned about a slightly higher incidence of intra-abdominal abscess, although it was not statistically significant [42]. This is one trend to monitor especially in cases with perforation and peritoneal soilage. LA is otherwise safe for perforated appendicitis [44].

Little additional data was available regarding LA for an appendiceal abscess. LA is regarded to be safe for children with some benefits [45; 46]. There are actually better paediatric instruments available now. Its safety in pregnancy can only be extrapolated from experience in other laparoscopic procedures, particularly chole-cystectomy and gynaecological procedures. Diagnostic laparoscopy is useful in pregnant women suspected to have appendicitis to locate the appendix and confirm diagnosis. Diagnostic laparoscopy is largely regarded to be superior to the wait-and-see approach in all categories of patients, especially in women in the childbearing age group. [47; 48].

Benefit to Patient

The meta-analyses have confirmed key advantages in reduction of wound infection (by 60 %) and faster postoperative recovery (by 35%).

There were also some benefits in terms of reduction in pain and hospital stay, albeit minimal. No new data for postoperative adhesions. Cosmesis is superior to the open procedure, especially with smaller trocars now available. In terms of cost effectiveness, hospital costs for LA in most centres remains higher, although this is partially offset by earlier return to work.

Special technical considerations

There is no significant change in the basic technique that uses three ports. Techniques using one or two ports, or those using 2-3 mm instruments, are not routine. Newer and better equipment such as ultrasonic dissectors is making LA easier and safer.

It must be emphasized that the whole appendix must be removed at the base to avoid residual appendicitis [49].

Training recommendations

No change from the 1994 recommendations. LA is a good starting point to train residents in basic laparoscopic technique.

Recommendations for the new millenium

All patients should have a diagnostic laparoscopy when diagnosis is in doubt.

This is superior to the wait-and-see attitude. The old adage "When in doubt, open up" should be modified to "When in doubt, put in a scope". If the appendix is inflamed, proceed to remove it laparoscopically.

If the appendix appears normal, search for another pathology. In the absence of an obvious pathology, remove the appendix.

If no other pathology is found, it is wiser to remove the appendix to avoid missing an early appendicitis and to avoid future confusion. In the presence of another well-defined pathology, treat the condition accordingly. Remove the appendix if there is a risk of future confusion with recurrent right iliac fossa pain (e.g. endometriosis) and when the appendectomy will not endanger the patient in any way.

LA is feasible in all patients diagnosed with uncomplicated acute appendicitis. It can also be applied to cases of complicated acute appendicitis if expertise is available.

References

(Ref. 1 – 6 relate to high-quality studies, which the original recommendations in 1994 were based on. Ref. 7 – 49 are mainly high-quality studies but also other reports published since then.)

1. Attwood SE, Hill AD, Murphy PG, Thornton J, Stephens RB (1992) A prospective randomized trial of laparoscopic versus open appendectomy. Surgery 112: 497-501.
2. Tate JJ, Dawson JW, Chung SC, Lau WY, Li AK (1993) Laparoscopic versus open appendicectomy: prospective randomised trial. Lancet 342: 633-637.
3. Frazee RC, Roberts JW, Symmonds RE, et al. (1994) A prospective randomized trial comparing open versus laparoscopic appendectomy. Ann Surg 219: 725-728; discussion 728-731.
4. Kum CK, Ngoi SS, Goh PM, Tekant Y, Isaac JR (1993) Randomized controlled trial comparing laparoscopic and open appendicectomy. Br J Surg 80: 1599-1600.
5. Hebebrand D, Troidl H, Spangenberger W, et al. (1994) Laparoskopische oder klassische Appendektomie? Eine prospektiv randomisierte Studie. Chirurg 65: 112-120.
6. de Wilde RL (1991) Goodbye to late bowel obstruction after appendicectomy [letter]. Lancet 338: 1012.
7. Bauwens K, Schwenk W, Böhm B, et al. (1998) Rekonvaleszenz und Arbeitsunfähigkeitsdauer nach laparoskopischer und konventioneller Appendektomie. Eine prospektiv-randomisierte Studie. Chirurg 69: 541-545.
8. Cox MR, McCall JL, Toouli J, et al. (1996) Prospective randomized comparison of open versus laparoscopic appendectomy in men. World J Surg 20: 263-266.
9. Hansen JB, Smithers BM, Schache D, et al. (1996) Laparoscopic versus open appendectomy: prospective randomized trial. World J Surg 20: 17-21.

10. Hart R, Rajgopal C, Plewes A, et al. (1996) Laparoscopic versus open appendectomy: a prospective randomized trial of 81 patients. Can J Surg 39: 457-462.
11. Heikkinen TJ, Haukipuro K, Hulkko A (1998) Cost-effective appendectomy. Open or laparoscopic? A prospective randomized study. Surg Endosc 12: 1204-1208.
12. Hellberg A, Rudberg C, Kullman E, et al. (1999) Prospective randomized multicentre study of laparoscopic versus open appendicectomy. Br J Surg 86: 48-53.
13. Henle KP, Beller S, Rechner J, et al. (1996) Laparoskopische versus konventionelle Appendektomie: Eine prospektive, randomisierte Studie. Chirurg 67: 526-530.
14. Kald A, Kullman E, Anderberg B, et al. (1999) Cost-minimisation analysis of laparoscopic and open appendicectomy. Eur J Surg 165: 579-582.
15. Kazemier G, de Zeeuw GR, Lange JF, Hop WCJ, Bonjer HJ (1997) Laparoscopic vs open appendectomy. A randomized clinical trial. Surg Endosc 11: 336-340.
16. Laine S, Rantala A, Gullichsen R, Ovaska J (1997) Laparoscopic appendectomy-is it worthwhile? A prospective, randomized study in young women. Surg Endosc 11: 95-97.
17. Lejus C, Delile L, Plattner V, et al. (1996) Randomized, single-blinded trial of laparoscopic versus open appendectomy in children: effects on postoperative analgesia. Anesthesiology 84: 801-806.
18. Macarulla E, Vallet J, Abad JM, et al. (1997) Laparoscopic versus open appendectomy: a prospective randomized trial. Surg Laparosc Endosc 7: 335-339.
19. Martin LC, Puente I, Sosa JL, et al. (1995) Open versus laparoscopic appendectomy. A prospective randomized comparison. Ann Surg 222: 256-261; discussion 261-252.
20. Minné L, Varner D, Burnell A, et al. (1997) Laparoscopic vs open appendectomy. Prospective randomized study of outcomes. Arch Surg 132: 708-711; discussion 712.
21. Mutter D, Vix M, Bui A, et al. (1996) Laparoscopy not recommended for routine appendectomy in men: results of a prospective randomized study. Surgery 120: 71-74.
22. Ortega AE, Hunter JG, Peters JH, et al. (1995) A prospective, randomized comparison of laparoscopic appendectomy with open appendectomy. Am J Surg 169: 208-213.
23. Reiertsen O, Larsen S, Trondsen E, et al. (1997) Randomized controlled trial with sequential design of laparoscopic versus conventional appendicectomy. Br J Surg 84: 842-847.
24. Sezeur A, Bure-Rossier AM, Rio D, et al. (1997) La coelioscopie augmente-t-elle le risque bactériologiuqe de l'appendicectomie? Résultats d'une étude prospective randomisée. Ann Chir 51: 243-247.
25. Williams MD, Collins JN, Wright TF, Fenoglio ME (1996) Laparoscopic versus open appendectomy. South Med J 89: 668-674.
26. Bannon MP, Zietlow SP, Harmsen WS, et al. (1997) Prospective randomized comparison of laparoscopic and open appendectomy [abstract]. Gastroenterology 112: A1429.
27. Meynaud-Kraemer L, Colin C, Vergnon P, Barth X (1999) Wound infection in open versus laparoscopic appendectomy. A meta-analysis. Int J Technol Assess Health Care 15: 380-391.
28. Esposito P, Cerbone D, Rotondano G, et al. (1997) Laparoscopic appendectomy: Our experience [abstract]. Gastrointest Endosc 45: Ab186.
29. Hoff C, Ruers T, Jakimowicz J (1995) Randomized study of laparoscopic versus open appendicectomy [abstract]. Surg Endosc 9: 605.
30. Loh A, Loosemore TM, Griffiths AB, Fiennes AGTW, Taylor RS, Less pain and earlier return to work after laparoscopic than after open appendicectomy: a randomized prospective study [abstract], 3rd World Congress of Endoscopic Surgery, Bordeaux, France, 1992.
31. May PJ, Laparoskopische versus konventionelle Appendektomie - eine prospektiv randomisierte Studie [M.D. thesis], RWTH Aachen, Aachen, 1997
32. Milewczyk M, Michalik M, Budzinski R (1998) Laparoscopic versus open appendectomy - a prospective, randomized, unicenter study [abstract]. Surg Endosc 12: 572.
33. Rohr S, Thiry CL, de Manzini N, Perrauid V, Meyer C (1994) Laparoscopic vs open appendectomy in men: a prospective randomized study [abstract]. Br J Surg 81(Suppl.): 6-7.
34. Stare R, Kocman I, Povsic Cevra Z, Zgrebec Z, Kovacic D, Results of a prospective randomised study of laparoscopic appendectomy in community hospital, 6th World Congress of Endoscopic Surgery, Rome, Italy, 1998.

35. Witten KI, Die chirurgische Behandlung der akuten Appendizitis. Ein Methodenvergleich zwischen laparoskopischer und konventioneller Appendektomie im Rahmen einer prospektiv randomisierten Studien an zweihundert Patienten [M.D. thesis], Georg-August-University, Göttingen, 2000
36. Yeung CK, Yip KF, Lee KH, Lau WY (1997) The role of minimally invasive surgery in the management of acute appendicitis in children: a prospective randomized trial of laparoscopic vs conventional appendectomy [abstract]. Asian J Surg 20: S55.
37. Navarra G, Ascanelli S, Turini A, Tonini G, Pozza E (2000) Laparoscopic versus open appendectomy in females with pain in right iliac fossa [abstract]. Surg Endosc 14(Suppl.1): S128.
38. Bruwer F, Coetzer M, Warren BL (2000) Early results of a randomized controlled study of laparoscopic vs open surgical exploration in pre-menopausal women with suspected acute appendicitis [abtsract]. Surg Endosc 14(Suppl.1): S110.
39. Sauerland S, Lefering R, Holthausen U, Neugebauer EAM (1998) Laparoscopic vs conventional appendectomy--a meta-analysis of randomised controlled trials. Langenbeck's Arch Surg 383: 289-295.
40. Garbutt JM, Soper NJ, Shannon WD, Botero A, Littenberg B (1999) Meta-analysis of randomized controlled trials comparing laparoscopic and open appendectomy. Surg Laparosc Endosc 9: 17-26.
41. Chung RS, Rowland DY, Li P, Diaz J (1999) A meta-analysis of randomized controlled trials of laparoscopic versus conventional appendectomy. Am J Surg 177: 250-256.
42. Golub R, Siddiqui F, Pohl D (1998) Laparoscopic versus open appendectomy: a metaanalysis. J Am Coll Surg 186: 545-553.
43. Temple LK, Litwin DE, McLeod RS (1999) A meta-analysis of laparoscopic versus open appendectomy in patients suspected of having acute appendicitis. Can J Surg 42: 377-383.
44. Khalili TM, Hiatt JR, Savar A, Lau C, Margulies DR (1999) Perforated appendicitis is not a contraindication to laparoscopy. Am Surg 65: 965-967.
45. Blakely ML, Spurbeck W, Lakshman S, Lobe TE (1998) Current status of laparoscopic appendectomy in children. Curr Opin Pediatr 10: 315-317.
46. Steyaert H, Hendrice C, Lereau L, et al. (1999) Laparoscopic appendectomy in children: sense or nonsense? Acta Chir Belg 99: 119-124.
47. Olsen JB, Myren CJ, Haahr PE (1993) Randomized study of the value of laparoscopy before appendicectomy. Br J Surg 80: 922-923.
48. Jadallah FA, Abdul-Ghani AA, Tibblin S (1994) Diagnostic laparoscopy reduces unnecessary appendicectomy in fertile women. Eur J Surg 160: 41-45.
49. Milne AA, Bradbury AW (1996) 'Residual' appendicitis following incomplete laparoscopic appendicectomy. Br J Surg 83: 217.

Laparoscopic hernia repair:

E.A.E.S. Consensus Development Conference (1997)[1,2] with updating comments (2000)

Conference organizers (1994):

A. FINGERHUT, Department of Surgery, Centre Hospitalier Intercommunal, Poissy (France);

A. PAUL, Surgical Clinic Merheim, 2nd Department of Surgery, University of Cologne (Germany);

E. NEUGEBAUER, Biochemical and Experimental Division, 2nd Department of Surgery, University of Cologne (Germany);

H. TROIDL, Surgical Clinic Merheim, 2nd Department of Surgery, University of Cologne (Germany);

E. EYPASCH, Surgical Clinic Merheim, 2nd Department of Surgery, University of Cologne (Germany);

C. K. KUM, Surgical Clinic Merheim, 2nd Department of Surgery, University of Cologne (Germany);

M. MISEREZ, Surgical Clinic Merheim, 2nd Department of Surgery, University of Cologne (Germany);

Expert Panel (1994):

J. H. ALEXANDRE, Department of Surgery, Hôpital Broussais Chirurgie II, Paris (France);

M. BÜCHLER, University Hospital for Visceral and Transplantation Surgery, Bern (Switzerland);

J. L. DULUCQ, Department of Surgery, M.S.P. Bagatelle, Talence- Bordeaux (France);

P. GO, Department of Surgery, University Hospital Maastricht, Maastricht (The Netherlands);

1) Held at the 2nd International Congress of the European Association for Endoscopic Surgery (E.A.E.S.), Madrid, Spain, 15-17 September, 1994
2) The original conference is published in Surg Endosc (1995) 9: 550-563.

J. HIMPENS, Department of Surgery, Algemeen Ziekenhuis St-Blasius, Dendermonde (Belgium);

CH. KLAIBER, Department of Surgery, Spital, Aarberg (Switzerland);

E. LAPORTE, Department of Surgery, Policlinica Teknon, Barcelona (Spain);

B. MILLAT, Department of Surgery, Hopital St Eloi (then La Peronie), Montpellier (France);

J. MOUIEL, Department of Digestive Surgery, Hopital Saint Roch, Nice (France);

L. NYHUS, Department of Surgery, College of Medicine, University of Illinois, Chicago (U.S.A.);

V. SCHUMPELICK, Department of Surgery, Clinic RWTH, Aachen (Germany)

Updating comments (2000):

A. FINGERHUT, Surgical Unit, Centre Hospitalier Intercommunal de Poissy-St Germain, Poissy (France);

B. MILLAT, Surgical Unit, Hôpital St Eloi, Montpellier (France);

N. BATAILLE, Surgical Unit, Centre Hospitalier Intercommunal de Poissy-St Germain, St Germain (France);

E. YACHOUCHI, Surgical Unit, Centre Hospitalier Intercommunal de Poissy-St Germain, Poissy (France);

C.DZIRI, Surgical Unit, Hôpital Charles Nicole, Tunis (Tunisia);

M.-J. BOUDET, Surgical Unit, Hôpital des Gardiens de la Paix, Paris (France) and Medicosurgical Department of Digestive Tract Pathology, IMM, Paris (France);

A. PAUL, Surgical Unit, University of Cologne, Cologne (Germany).

Consensus statements (1994)

Question 1. Is there a need for the classification of groin hernias, and if so, which classification should be used?

Several classifications for groin hernias have been proposed (Alexandre, Bendavid, Gilbert, Nyhus, Schumpelick). The majority of the panelists refer to Nyhus' classification (Table 1). It is suggested to apply this classification in future trials. However, the accuracy and reproducibility of any classification in laparoscopic hernia repair still has to be demonstrated.

In any case, the minimal requirements for future studies are classifications which accurately describe the defects:

- the type: direct, indirect, femoral or combined
- state of the internal ring (dilated or not)
- presence and size of the posterior wall defect
- size and contents of the sac
- whether primary or recurrent

Table 1: Nyhus classification for groin hernia (taken from [1])

Type of Hernia	Anatomical defect
I	Indirect hernia - normal internal ring
II	Indirect hernia - dilated internal ring
III A	Direct hernia - posterior wall defect
III B	Large indirect hernia - posterior wall defect
III C	Femoral hernia
IV	Recurrent hernia

Question 2. In what stage of technology assessment is endoscopic hernia repair in September 1994?

Endoscopic hernia repair is presently a **feasible** alternative for conventional hernia repair if performed by **experienced** endoscopic surgeons. It appears to be **efficacious** in the **short-term**. It has **not yet** reached the **effectiveness** stage in **general practice**. Detailed analysis on **cost-effectiveness** and **cost-benefits** are lacking. Although some aspects of endoscopic hernia repair are very promising (e.g. recurrence and bilateral hernia), it cannot be considered the standard treatment.

Question 3. Is endoscopic hernia repair safe?

Endoscopic hernia repair might be as safe as the open procedure. However, up until now, safety aspects have not been sufficiently evaluated. Most panelists agreed that it has the same potential for serious complications as in open surgery, such as post-operative ileus, nerve injury, and injuries to large vessels. Reporting all complications, fatal or not, are encouraged and necessary for further evaluation.

Question 4. Is endoscopic hernia repair beneficial to the patient?

The potential reduction in the incidence of hematoma and clinically relevant wound infections has yet to be proven. Postoperative pain seems to be diminished. Although it seems to allow earlier return to normal activities, post-operative disability and hospital stay are highly dependent on activity, motivation and social status of the patient as well as on the structure of the health care system.

Objective measurement (e.g. standardized exercise tests) should be developed and used to evaluate return to normal activity. As in other endoscopic procedures, there is a potential for better cosmetic results. The long-term recurrence rate for endoscopic hernia repair is not known.

Question 5. Who are potential candidates for endoscopic hernia repair?

Candidates:
- types III A-C
- recurrences (type IV), bilateral hernia
- type II?

Contra-indications:

Absolute:
- high risk patients for general anesthesia or conventional surgery
- uncorrected bleeding disorders
- proven adverse reaction to foreign material
- major intra-abdominal disease (e.g. ascites)

Relative:
- incarcerated or scrotal (sliding) hernia
- young age (sac resection only)
- prior major abdominal operations

Question 6. What are the concepts for future evaluation of endoscopic hernia repair?

There is a definite need for classification and randomized controlled (multicenter) trials with clear endpoints:

- complication and recurrence rates (clinical follow-up >5 years, with <5% lost to follow-up)
  - pain and resumption of physical activity
  - size, type and route of mesh placement

Endoscopic techniques should be compared to conventional hernia or open pre-peritoneal prosthetic mesh repair techniques vs. laparoscopic transabdominal preperitoneal (TAPP) and/or totally extraperitoneal (TEP) (sometimes also called totally preperitoneal repair (TPP)).

Question 7. Should endoscopic hernia repair be performed outside clinical trials?

In 1994, we recommend that endoscopic hernia repair should only be performed after appropriate training and with some sort of quality control, and should be restricted to participation in clinical trials.

Updating comments (2000)

Introduction

When in 1994 the E.A.E.S. consensus development conference (CDC) was held on the then new laparoscopic hernia repair, there were only two randomized trials available for analysis [2; 3]. Today, there are more than 60, with more than 12500 patients entered. Therefore updated answers to the 7 original questions are presented herein.

Methodology

Through a systemic review of the literature (Medline), completed by hand search with cross-referencing, we found that, of the 62 studies analyzed, nine lacked homogeneity (i.e. the techniques and the suture or repair material used were modified in such a way that comparisons were impossible, even though the names of the operations were apparently the same), patient populations were mixed (e.g. males and females), follow-up was not provided or was insufficient (less than 3 or 5 years, and the number of patients lost to follow-up was above 10% or not given, follow-up method was by telephone, mail response or information was not given) in 24, valid endpoints (many papers did not have recurrence as their main endpoint) were not provided in 25, and 47 of these (negative) studies lacked sufficient power. Just as an example, to show that the recurrence rate can be lowered from

5% to 3% with such and such technique, with an alpha level set at 5% and a beta level at 10% (90% power), no less than 736 patients would be required!

Question 1. Is there a need for a classification of groin hernias, and if so, which classification should be used?

The Nyhus classification (**Table 1**, [1]) was – and still is – the most widely known and used. Two modifications were proposed in order to classify the size and the contents of the sac. Nevertheless, in predicting the intraoperative Nyhus hernia type, clinical examination and ultrasonography have only moderate sensitivity and specificity (61% and 57%; 54% and 43% respectively [4]).

Question 2. At what stage of technology assessment is laparoscopic hernia repair?

Hernia repair had already been shown to be feasible in 1994, but essentially by those pioneer laparoscopic surgeons who became experienced in the new field. Laparoscopic hernia repair was considered to be efficacious in the short-term, but not yet effective in overall general practice. In the current literature, laparoscopic hernia repair is considered a difficult procedure and is not widely practiced (Table 2).

Table 2: The acceptance of laparoscopic inguinal hernia repair throughout Europe

Country, Year	Number of total cases	% laparoscopy
Switzerland, 1994 [5]	1118 recurrent repairs	5%
North-Rhine, Germany, 1995 [6]	19527 primary repairs	6.7%
Sweden, 1996 [7]	4056 primary repairs	11% (TAPP) 10% (TEP)
Netherlands, 1995 [8]	448 surveyed surgeons	1.6%
West of Scotland, 1999 [9]	3400 primary repairs	3.6%

Cost-effectiveness and cost-benefit studies were considered to be lacking in 1994. Today, of two known studies [10; 11], only one [10] seems satisfactory: 200 male patients were randomized to either the laparoscopic transabdominal preperitoneal or Shouldice repairs. The laparoscopic repair took 10 min longer (p=0.009). There were no statistically significant differences found either in duration of hospital stay or complication rates. The time off work was found to be statistically significantly shorter among the working population only. The conclusion of this study was that laparoscopic hernia repair should be for the young, working population only.

When compared with the open hernia repair technique, laparoscopic hernia repair was found to be between 1.41 [2] and 17 [12] times more expensive than the open repair techniques. Only two studies [13; 14], the latter [14] reporting on direct and indirect costs, concluded that laparoscopic repair was less expensive (when they were considered in their global economical setting).

Question 3. Is laparoscopic hernia repair safe?

In 1994, this was unanswered. The jury felt that laparoscopic repair had the same potential for complications as open surgery. In addition, however, there was the possibility of post-operative obstruction, nerve injuries, and of course, intestinal and large vessel injuries whether during dissection, but above all, when inserting the trocars at the beginning of operation.

Complications were reported in about 90% of the studies. The overall complication rates ranged from 12% [15] to 17% [16], but the definitions of complications varied greatly from one report to another. Serious, life-threatening complications were seemingly rare. However, it is unfortunately, well known, that serious and life-loss generating complications are rarely, if ever, reported in series on hernia repair. As well, conversions were withdrawn from analysis in more than 30% of the studies, some of which were for complications.

The true incidence of infection is probably very difficult to assess. The reasons for this are multiple. First, the infection rate is already very low in clean operations [17], and lowest for inguinal hernia repair [18]. Infection after open mesh repair has been reported to be between 0.09% for all types of (open) mesh repair [9] and 0.3% for the tension-free Lichtenstein type repair [19]. The prevalence of infection in laparoscopic hernia (mesh) repair ranges from 2/1139 (0.2%) [20] to 3/500 (0.6%) [21] when no prophylactic antibiotics are given. Second, one of the attributes of laparoscopic surgery is to allow the patient to leave the hospital earlier. Estimates have been made that at least two of three infections become apparent only once the patient has left the hospital [22]. Infection is an ever present and important problem. Not only does it increase hospital stay when discovered in hospital, but also it is responsible for further visits, further treatment and therefore, further costs.

Moreover, as infection is implicated in recurrence, this is equally a reason for further discomfort and costs. Up to 50% of recurrences have been found to be associated with infection [23], while 33% of infected hernias result in recurrence [24].

Question 4. Is laparoscopic hernia repair beneficial to the patient?

In a study published in 1992, Wright et al. [25] compared the early outcome of 60 patients undergoing open with 60 patients undergoing totally extraperitoneal

(TEP) laparoscopic repair of inguinal hernia. They found a significant difference in hospital stay in favor of the laparoscopic technique (2 vs. 1 days, p<0.05). However, both the median duration of anesthesia and of operation (in minutes) were significantly longer in the laparoscopic arm (60 (53-72) versus 80 (70-90) (p<0.0001) for anesthesia, and 45 (35-52) versus 58 (46-69)(p<0.0001), for surgery, respectively. Laparoscopic inguinal hernia repair is reported to cause less pain. Mixter et al. [26] performed a prospective controlled study of repair in 94 hernias (70 patients) received oral ibuprofen (800 mg) 1 h before vs. IV intraoperative ketorolac 60 mg.. Although the laparoscopic technique was not described (was it a transabdominal preperitoneal (TAPP) or TEP repair?), there was no statistically significant difference found in the number of patients requiring postoperative narcotics or in visual analogue scores (VAS). This shows that pain is probably not the best criteria to judge on. Effective pain relief can and should be given adequately to all patients: no patient should have postoperative pain. A measure of the amount of painkillers necessary to obtain complete relief seems more appropriate. As well, progress in pain relief has made it obvious that different types of pain killers are necessary according to whether the peritoneal cavity has been violated or not, so that comparisons of two techniques (TAPP and TEP, for instance) with the same analgesic are not proper. Last, even if one can show that there is statistically less postoperative pain [27] in laparoscopic hernia repair, the main question is whether the difference between one or two pain killer capsules has any clinical relevance!

According to Cunningham et al. [28], persistent pain (10% of patients at 2 years) is more frequent in patients without palpable hernia preoperatively, those who experience postoperative anesthesia or pain, who stay off work longer, irrespective of type of hernia or repair. For these authors, the origin of pain is the periosteal sutures.

Return to work is not a good criterion as social and economical factors intervene more than technique and therefore probably skew any evaluation. As well, the definition of "return to work" or "return to normal activities" varies so widely from one country to another (as can be seen in **Table 3**), that these numbers cannot be used for effective comparisons from one series to another.

Table 3: Return to work after open and laparoscopic hernia repair

Author, year	Comparison groups with number of cases	Result	P-Value
Liem [27]	507 surgeon's preference vs. 487 TEP	10 vs. 6d	p < 0.001
Lorentz	445 Shouldice vs. 448 TAPP	65 vs. 35d	p < 0.001
Stoker [3]	75 darn vs. 75 TAPP	28 vs. 14d	p < 0.001
Heikkinen [29]	18 Lichtenstein vs. 20 TAPP	19 vs. 14d	p < 0.03

Whereas some studies [3; 27; 29] found a statistically significant difference in duration of lay off of work, others [13; 15; 30-32] did not find any differences. When reporting this endpoint, however, the percentage of patients who are normally at work should be mentioned. According to one report, only 47% of patients are at their usual job at time of operation [33]. As well, the motivation to return to normal activities, whether it is reported as a return to work or not, is dependent on the type of insurance or workers compensation the patient has. In one paper on open repair, those patients with worker's compensation returned to work later than those who did not have any [34].

The problem of cosmesis has given rise to very few publications favoring the laparoscopic technique over the open technique. In fact, one can question the validity of such a criteria in hernia repair as the incision in open repair can be placed low and horizontal, therefore with little if any cosmetic prejudice. Not withstanding, the literature does not allow any conclusions in one direction or the other.

Although the relevance of recurrence as the main endpoint has been questioned, in our opinion, this should be the case for several reasons : 1) A "lump" or "bulge" in the groin is the main symptom of which the patient complains initially [15; 35; 36] as well as, often, when the hernia recurs. 2) 10 % of all hernia operations in the USA are for recurrence [35; 37], and all reported series on hernia repair include 5 to 18% of recurrent hernia (figure 3); 3) Operation for recurrence is a more difficult operation, with increased risk of permanent cord and nerve damage. As the orifice of recurrent, more long standing hernia, is often fibrotic, strangulation might have more severe consequences. 4) Recurrence is the only complication of hernia that has potentially life-threatening consequences. 5) Last, there is an increased risk of re-recurrence as the re-recurrence rate can be as high as 39% [19; 38]. Recurrence is therefore responsible for increased morbidity, convalescence, longer periods of time of incomfort and lay-off from work before operation as well as longer duration of time before return to full activity or work, and above all, for all these mentioned reasons, recurrence leads to increased costs [10].

In the 20 studies on laparoscopic surgery in which the follow-up was given, only 8 of the studies reported that less than 10% of their patients were lost to follow-up. In these series, however, the median of follow-up ranged from 1-20 months. With a median follow-up of 607 days and 3% of patients lost to follow-up, the series reported by Liem et al. [27] is an example for all.

Table 4: Recurrence rates

Author, year	Recurrences	
Maddern, 1994 [16]	7/101	(7%)
Payne, 1994 [2]	8/110	(7.3%)
Stoker, 1994 [3]	19/167	(11.4%)
Wilson, 1995 [39]	30/242	(12.5%)
Vogt, 1995 [40]	16/65	(24.5%)

Question 5. Who are the potential candidates for laparoscopic hernia repair?

In 1994, the participants of the consensus conference thought that Nyhus Type I and II hernias as well as hernia in the child should not undergo laparoscopic repair. Patients with Nyhus types III A, B and C, recurrences (type IV), or bilateral hernia could most likely benefit from this technique.

Are bilateral and/or recurrent hernia a good indication for laparoscopic repair? Although the results reported originated from sub-group analysis on repair of recurrent hernia, Champault et al found that the Stoppa repair was associated with less re-recurrence than the laparoscopic technique [41]. Only one study has studied this point specifically [42]. The authors compared 37 patients with 52 recurrent hernias operated on with the Stoppa technique to 42 patients with 56 recurrent hernias operated on with the TAPP technique. Although there were more complications such as infected wounds, more postoperative pain, and later return to work in the Stoppa group, the number of re-recurrences was less at 12 months (1/52 = 1.9% versus 7/56 = 12.5%; p = 0.04) in the laparoscopic arm. Overall costs did not differ significantly.

In 1994, the participants in the consensus conference thought that absolute contra-indications to laparoscopic hernia repair should include patients with…

- …a high risk for general anesthesia
- …uncorrected bleeding disorders
- …proven adverse reaction to foreign material
- …major intra-abdominal disease (e.g. ascites).

The relative contra-indications included incarcerated or large scrotal (sliding) hernia, young age in which resection of sac only is required, and previous major abdominal operations (for the TAPP repairs). Today, nothing much has been written to support or to refute these limitations, but the threshold for laparoscopic surgery, in general, has decreased considerably since 1994.

Question 6. What are the concepts for future evaluation of laparoscopic hernia repair?

In 1994, the jury felt that there was a definite need for adequate classification and randomized controlled (multicenter) trials to compare laparoscopic hernia repair versus conventional hernia repair (herniorrhaphy), and also versus open preperitoneal mesh (tension-free) repair. Clear end-points are needed: complication and recurrence rates (at 5 years), with < 5% of patients lost to follow-up, post-operative (permanent) pain, resumption of physical activity as evaluated by tests as opposed to the date of subjective resumption of "normal" activity. As seen above, few if any of the reported studies [27] have responded to this.

Question 7. Should laparoscopic hernia repair be performed outside clinical trials?

The participants in the 1994 jury said "no", this technique should probably not be routinely performed until appropriate data were available. Appropriate data are still lacking; yet 1.5-21% of surgeons perform hernia repair laparoscopically today [5-9]. Following is the evaluation of the strength of evidence at the time of the conference in 1994 and the current literature assessment (**Table 5**):

Table 5: Stages of technology assessment in endoscopic hernia repair

Stages in technology assessment	In 1994...	...and 2000
1. Feasibility (Technical performance, applicability, safety, complications, morbidity, mortality)	I	III
2. Efficacy (Benefit for the patient demonstrated in centers of excellence)	II	III
3. Effectiveness (Benefit for the patient under normal clinical conditions, i.e., good results reproducible with widespread application)	0	II
4. Efficiency (Benefit in terms of costs)	0	Certainly not
5. Gold Standard	No	No

References

(Ref. 1 – 3 relate to high-quality studies, which the original recommendations in 1994 were based on. Ref. 4 – 42 are mainly high-quality studies but also other reports published since then.)

1. Nyhus LM, Klein MS, Rogers FB (1991) Inguinal hernia. Curr Probl Surg 28: 401-450.
2. Payne JH, Jr., Grininger LM, Izawa MT, et al. (1994) Laparoscopic or open inguinal herniorrhaphy? A randomized prospective trial. Arch Surg 129: 973-981.
3. Stoker DL, Spiegelhalter DJ, Singh R, Wellwood JM (1994) Laparoscopic versus open inguinal hernia repair: randomised prospective trial. Lancet 343: 1243-1245.
4. Renzulli P, Frei E, Schäfer M, et al. (1997) Preoperative Nyhus classification of inguinal hernias and type-related individual hernia repair. A case for diagnostic laparoscopy. Surg Laparosc Endosc 7: 373-377.
5. Herzog U, Kocher T (1996) Leistenhernienchirurgie in der Schweiz 1994. Eine Umfrage an 142 Ausbildungskliniken in der Schweiz. Chirurg 67: 921-926.
6. Schumpelick V, Arlt G, Steinau G (1997) Leistenhernien bei Erwachsenen und Kindern. Dt Ärztebl 94: A-3268-3276.
7. Nilsson E, Haapaniemi S, Gruber G, Sandblom G (1998) Methods of repair and risk for reoperation in Swedish hernia surgery from 1992 to 1996. Br J Surg 85: 1686-1691.
8. Simons MP, Hoitsma HF, Mullan FJ (1995) Primary inguinal hernia repair in The Netherlands. Eur J Surg 161: 345-348.

9. Taylor SG, O'Dwyer PJ (1999) Chronic groin sepsis following tension-free inguinal hernioplasty. Br J Surg 86: 562-565.

10. Kald A, Anderberg B, Carlsson P, Park PO, Smedh K (1997) Surgical outcome and cost-minimisation-analyses of laparoscopic and open hernia repair: a randomised prospective trial with one year follow up. Eur J Surg 163: 505-510.

11. Damamme A, Samama G, D'Alche-Gautier MJ, et al. (1998) Evaluation médico-économique de la cure de hernie inguinale: Shouldice vs laparoscopie. Ann Chir 52: 11-16.

12. Zieren J, Zieren HU, Jacobi CA, Wenger FA, Müller JM (1998) Prospective randomized study comparing laparoscopic and open tension-free inguinal hernia repair with Shouldice's operation. Am J Surg 175: 330-333.

13. Barkun JS, Wexler MJ, Hinchey EJ, Thibeault D, Meakins JL (1995) Laparoscopic versus open inguinal herniorrhaphy: preliminary results of a randomized controlled trial. Surgery 118: 703-710.

14. Liem MS, Halsema JA, van der Graaf Y, et al. (1997) Cost-effectiveness of extraperitoneal laparoscopic inguinal hernia repair: a randomized comparison with conventional herniorrhaphy. Ann Surg 226: 668-676.

15. Lawrence K, McWhinnie D, Goodwin A, et al. (1995) Randomised controlled trial of laparoscopic versus open repair of inguinal hernia: early results. BMJ 311: 981-985.

16. Maddern GJ, Rudkin G, Bessell JR, Devitt P, Ponte L (1994) A comparison of laparoscopic and open hernia repair as a day surgical procedure. Surg Endosc 8: 1404-1408.

17. The Southern Surgeons Club (1991) A prospective analysis of 1518 laparoscopic cholecystectomies. N Engl J Med 324: 1073-1078.

18. Rotman N, Hay JM, Lacaine F, Fagniez PL (1989) Prophylactic antibiotherapy in abdominal surgery. First- vs third-generation cephalosporins. Arch Surg 124: 323-327.

19. Shulman AG, Amid PK, Lichtenstein IL (1992) The safety of mesh repair for primary inguinal hernias: results of 3,019 operations from five diverse surgical sources. Am Surg 58: 255-257.

20. Fuchsjäger N, Feichter A, Kux M (1995) Die Lichtenstein-Plug-Methode zur Reparation von Rezidivleistenhernine. Indikation, Technik und Ergebnisse. Chirurg 66: 409-412.

21. Hofbauer C, Andersen PV, Juul P, Qvist N (1998) Late mesh rejection as a complication to transabdominal preperitoneal laparoscopic hernia repair. Surg Endosc 12: 1164-1165.

22. Hyryla ML, Sintonen H (1994) The use of health services in the management of wound infection. J Hosp Infect 26: 1-14.

23. Abrahamson J (1998) Etiology and pathophysiology of primary and recurrent groin hernia formation. Surg Clin North Am 78: 953-972.

24. Lowham AS, Filipi CJ, Fitzgibbons RJ, Jr., et al. (1997) Mechanisms of hernia recurrence after preperitoneal mesh repair. Traditional and laparoscopic. Ann Surg 225: 422-431.

25. Wright DM, Kennedy A, Baxter JN, et al. (1996) Early outcome after open versus extraperitoneal endoscopic tension-free hernioplasty: a randomized clinical trial. Surgery 119: 552-557.

26. Mixter CG, 3rd, Meeker LD, Gavin TJ (1998) Preemptive pain control in patients having laparoscopic hernia repair: a comparison of ketorolac and ibuprofen. Arch Surg 133: 432-437.

27. Liem MS, van der Graaf Y, van Steensel CJ, et al. (1997) Comparison of conventional anterior surgery and laparoscopic surgery for inguinal-hernia repair. N Engl J Med 336: 1541-1547.

28. Cunningham J, Temple WJ, Mitchell P, et al. (1996) Cooperative hernia study. Pain in the postrepair patient. Ann Surg 224: 598-602.

29. Heikkinen T, Haukipuro K, Leppala J, Hulkko A (1997) Total costs of laparoscopic and Lichtenstein inguinal hernia repairs: a randomized prospective study. Surg Laparosc Endosc 7: 1-5.

30. Wellwood J, Sculpher MJ, Stoker D, et al. (1998) Randomised controlled trial of laparoscopic versus open mesh repair for inguinal hernia: outcome and cost. BMJ 317: 103-110.

31. Bessell JR, Baxter P, Riddell P, Watkin S, Maddern GJ (1996) A randomized controlled trial of laparoscopic extraperitoneal hernia repair as a day surgical procedure. Surg Endosc 10: 495-500.
32. Schrenk P, Woisetschläger R, Rieger R, Wayand W (1996) Prospective randomized trial comparing postoperative pain and return to physical activity after transabdominal preperitoneal, total preperitoneal or Shouldice technique for inguinal hernia repair. Br J Surg 83: 1563-1566.
33. Burney RE, Jones KR, Coon JW, et al. (1997) Core outcomes measures for inguinal hernia repair. J Am Coll Surg 185: 509-515.
34. Salcedo-Wasicek MC, Thirlby RC (1995) Postoperative course after inguinal herniorrhaphy. A case-controlled comparison of patients receiving workers' compensation vs patients with commercial insurance. Arch Surg 130: 29-32.
35. Rutkow IM (1995) The recurrence rate in hernia surgery. How important is it? Arch Surg 130: 575-577.
36. Kingsnorth AN, Gray MR, Nott DM (1992) Prospective randomized trial comparing the Shouldice technique and plication darn for inguinal hernia. Br J Surg 79: 1068-1070.
37. Lichtenstein IL, Shulman AG, Amid PK, The tension-free repair of groin hernias. In: L.M. Nyhus (Ed.), Hernia, Lippincott, Philadelphia, 1995, pp. 237-249.
38. Glassow F (1976) Inguinal hernia repair. A comparison of the Shouldice and Cooper ligament repair of the posterior inguinal wall. Am J Surg 131: 306-311.
39. Wilson MS, Deans GT, Brough WA (1995) Prospective trial comparing Lichtenstein with laparoscopic tension-free mesh repair of inguinal hernia. Br J Surg 82: 274-277.
40. Vogt DM, Curet MJ, Pitcher DE, Martin DT, Zucker KA (1995) Preliminary results of a prospective randomized trial of laparoscopic onlay versus conventional inguinal herniorrhaphy. Am J Surg 169: 84-90.
41. Champault GG, Rizk N, Catheline JM, Turner R, Boutelier P (1997) Inguinal hernia repair: totally preperitoneal laparoscopic approach versus Stoppa operation: randomized trial of 100 cases. Surg Laparosc Endosc 7: 445-450.
42. Beets GL, Dirksen CD, Go PMNYH, et al. (1999) Open or laparoscopic preperitoneal mesh repair for recurrent inguinal hernia? A randomized controlled trial. Surg Endosc 13: 323-327.

Laparoscopic cholecystectomy:

E.A.E.S. Consensus Development Conference (1997)[1,2] with updating comments (2000)

Conference organizers (1994):

J. Périssat, Centre de Chirurgie, Université de Bordeaux, Bordeaux (France);

W. Wayand, 2nd Department of Surgery, General Hospital, Linz (Austria);

E. Neugebauer, Biochemical and Experimental Division, 2nd Department of Surgery, University of Cologne (Germany);

H. Troidl, Surgical Clinic Merheim, 2nd Department of Surgery, University of Cologne (Germany);

C. K. Kum, Department of Surgery, National University Hospital, Singapore (Singapore);

M. Miserez, Surgical Clinic Merheim, 2nd Department of Surgery, University of Cologne (Germany);

A. Paul, Surgical Clinic Merheim, 2nd Department of Surgery, University of Cologne (Germany);

Expert Panel (1994):

A. Cuschieri, Department of Surgery, Ninewells Hospital & Medical School, University of Dundee, Dundee, Scotland (U.K.);

T. C. Dupont, Jefe del Opto de Cirugia, Hospital Universitario Virgen del Rocio, Sevilla (Spain);

M. Garcia-Caballero, Department of Surgery, Medical Faculty, Malaga (Spain);

J. F. Gigot, Department de Chirurgie Digestive, St. Luc Hospital, Bruxelles (Belgique);

H. Glise, Department of Surgery, Norra Älsborgs, Länssjukhus-NAL, Trollhättan (Sweden);

C. Liguory, CMC Alma, Paris (France);

---

1) Held at the 2nd International Congress of the European Association for Endoscopic Surgery (E.A.E.S.), Madrid, Spain, 15-17 September, 1994

2) The original conference is published in Surg Endosc (1995) 9: 550-563.

M. MORINO, Surgical Clinic, University of Torino, Torino (Italy);
M. ROTHMUND, Department of Surgery, University of Marburg, Marburg (Germany);

Updating comments (2000):

W. WAYAND, 2nd Department of Surgery, General Hospital, Linz (Austria);
S. SAUERLAND, Biochemical and Experimental Division, 2nd Department of Surgery, University of Cologne (Germany)

Consensus statements (1994)

Question 1. What stage of technological development is laparoscopic cholecystectomy (LC) at (in Sept. 1994)?

LC is the procedure of choice for symptomatic uncomplicated cholelithiasis. As it is not possible to conduct randomized trials on LC vs open surgery anymore, it is important for all surgeons to audit continually the results of LC. Results of analyses on its cost effectiveness and cost benefits are dependent on the health care system. Open cholecystectomy remains the standard for comparison.

Question 2. Who should undergo LC?

1. The indications for cholecystectomy remain unchanged. LC is indicated for patients who are able to tolerate general anaesthesia without undue risk. It is also indicated in patients with calcified (porcelain) gallbladders.
2. Asymptomatic cholelithiases, in general, do not warrant cholecystectomy. Most of the patients remain asymptomatic. It is also rare for complications to occur without symptoms appearing first. Patients with symptomless gallstones that should be followed up closely include:
    i. Diabetics
    ii. Those with sickle cell disease
    iii. Children
    iv. Those on long-term somatostatin
    v. Those on immunosuppressive drugs
3. In the following conditions, LC is usually contraindicated.
    i. Generalized peritonitis
    ii. Septic shock from cholangitis
    iii. Severe acute pancreatitis
    iv. Cirrhosis with portal hypertension
    v. Severe coagulopathy that is not corrected
    vi. Cholecysto-enteric fistula
4. Extreme caution should be taken in the following groups of patients.
    i. Severe associated cardiorespiratory diseases
    ii. Previous upper abdominal surgery
    iii. Acute cholecystitis
    iv. Symptomatic cholecystitis in the second trimester of pregnancy
    These cases should be performed only by an experienced team.

Question 3. Is LC safe and feasible?

1. The incidence of common bile duct injury is still slightly higher than open surgery. Vascular injury and bowel injury are specific to LC. This is due to surgeon inexperience, limitations of the twodimensional view, lack of tactile sensation, and extension of indication to more difficult cases. Adequate training with close supervision and strict accreditation is required.
2. Operation time is similar or longer than the open procedure.
3. Morbidity from wound complications and postoperative recovery period are reduced with LC.
4. Mortality risk is similar.
5. In pregnant women, the risk of CO_2 pneumoperitoneum on the fetus in the first trimester is not fully known. LC in the third trimester should be avoided as it is technically difficult and carries a risk of injuring the uterus. Only in the second trimester is LC relatively safe, but it should only be performed by experienced operators in severely symptomatic or complicated cholelithiasis.
6. For acute cholecystitis, publications of data on small numbers of patients by keen endoscopic surgeons have reported complication rates not more than routine LC, even when performed in the same admission. However, the true safety cannot be known until more data are available. The threshold for conversion should be low. Indications for conversion include:
    i. Unclear anatomy
    ii. Gangrenous, friable gallbladder that is difficult to handle
    iii. bleeding
    iv. technical problems
    v. unduly long operation with no progress

Question 4. Is it beneficial to the patients?

1. LC leads to markedly less postoperative pain, shorter hospital stay, earlier return to normal activities, and better cosmesis.
2. In general, LC has a distinct advantage over open cholecystectomy.

Question 5. How should common bile stones be managed?

- This question has been answered separately in 1997. Please refer to the relevant chapter of this book! –

Question 6. What are the special technical aspects to be considered during LC?

1. If problems are encountered during CO_2 insufflation with the Veres needle, the open technique should be used.

2. The junction between the cystic duct and the gallbladder must always be clearly defined. Dissection of the junction between the cystic duct and the CBD is not necessary. Dissection in this area, principally done to identify the CBD, is, however, associated with the risk of inadvertent damage to the CBD itself.

3. Coagulation in Calot's triangle should be kept to a minimum. If needed, either bipolar or soft monopolar (< 200 mV) coagulation is preferred.

4. Either metal clips (at least two) or locking clips are safe for securing the cystic artery and duct. In event of a large cystic duct, a ligature is safer.

5. The prevention of CBD damage by routine intraoperative cholangiogram (IOC) is not proven. However, IOC allows immediate detection of the injury and thus primary repair with better prognosis. IOC should be done when

    i. anatomy is not well seen;

    ii. duct injury is suspected;

    iii. common bile duct stones are suspected.

    All surgeons should be trained to perform IOC.

6. To avoid injury to the CBD, the following principles should be adhered to:

    i. Unambiguously identify the structures in Calot's triangle

    ii. Avoid unnecessary coagulation

    iii. Dissect starting from the gallbladder-cystic duct junction

    iv. Perform IOC when the anatomy is not clear

    v. Convert to open surgery when in doubt

7. Drainage is usually not required.

8. Suturing of trocar sites 10 mm or more is recommended especially when such a site has been dilated or extended for extraction of the gallbladder.

Question 7. What are the training recommendations for LC?

Refer to E.A.E.S. guidelines published in Surgical Endoscopy 1994; 8: 721-722.

Updating comments (2000)

Introduction

When in 1994 the EAES consensus panelists met for discussion, laparoscopic cholecystectomy (LC) had been evaluated in just 4 RCTs until then [1-4], and the panelists feared that future trials were already impossible due to the "distinct advantage" of LC.

Two years later, however, after an extensive and detailed analysis of all evidence available by end of 1994, Sara H. Downs and her colleagues concluded on the basis of 15 RCTs [1-21] that, "surgeons should not be encouraged to replace mini-chole-cystectomy with laparoscopic cholecystectomy" [22].

The most important piece of new information, however, was provided by the first blinded trial on the comparison of mini-laparotomy cholecystectomy (MC) and LC, which was published by Majeed and coworkers in 1996 [19; 20]. The MC approach is defined as a 5-7 cm subcostal or right paramedian incision The Majeed trial has most elegantly shown that much of the benefit of LC can be explained by self-fulfilling optimistic expectations from carers and patients. Nevertheless, LC (and not MC) has become the standard procedure for cholecystolithiasis all over the world.

After the Majeed trial, scientific interest in LC has shifted away from the compa-rison between laparoscopic and open or mini-lap cholecystectomy to more detailled aspects of therapy. Issues that have been investigated in randomized clinical trial include various refinements in surgical technique, such as reusable instruments [23], 5 mm instruments [24], transumbilical access [25], ultrasonically activated shears [26], three-dimensional imaging [27], low- or no-pressure pneumoperito-neum [28-30], humidified [31] and preheated insufflation gas [32; 33].

New trials that compared LC versus OC or MC, reported clinical results only sparingly. Most of them assessed the pathophysiological benefits of minimally inva-sive surgery with regard to postoperative immune function [34], pulmonary func-tion [35-37], heamostasis [38], and endocrine stress response [39; 40].. Many more trials have been undertaken to investigate the various modalities of pain treatment (see [41] for an overview). In consequence, many details of LC have been further clarified within many rigorous investigations.

Question 1. What stage of technological development is LC at (in 2000)?

The 1994 statement is true without change: LC is the procedure of choice for symptomatic uncomplicated cholelithiasis.

Question 2. Who should undergo LC?

Today, as compared to 1994, the indications for LC are seen more widely:

■ Even asymptomatic patients may benefit from LC, if they have risk factors that unambigiously predict future symptoms or complications, for instance in a young, obese, fair-haired female, in whom several pregancies during life and a life span of 60 years are likely.

■ In patients with severe associated cardiorespiratory diseases a reduction of intraabdominal pressure can reduce haemodynamic stress [42] and hepatic dys-function [43] during and after LC. Gasless LC may turn out even better [44], so that these patients no longer can be denied laparoscopy.

■ In cases with acute cholecystitis, early cholecystectomy has been shown to be more effective than delayed surgery [45]. New evidence suggests that LC is safe to perform in such cases, although a high conversion rate must be anticipated [46].

■ Patients with cholecysto-enteric fistulae may also undergo LC. Most of these fistulae are detected only intraoperatively during LC, and there is no need for an experienced surgeon to convert these cases to open surgery.

Question 3. Is LC safe and feasible?

The fear in 1994, that common bile duct injury is more likely to occur during LC, has generally been confirmed, although the importance of this problem is still under debate. Populations-based data indicate, that this increase in complication rates partly settles down, when the learning curve for LC has passed [47-49].

Question 4. Is it beneficial to the patients?

In 2000, it is without doubt that LC is superior to OC. However, if compared against MC, the benefits of LC may be much smaller. Here again, the Sheffield trial is a milestone in evaluating the comparative effectiveness of LC [19].

Question 6. What are the special technical aspects to be considered during LC?

It is impossible to summarize all the technical modifications of LC that have been proposed and evaluated during the last years. Evidence from RCTs is available to suggest the following intraoperative procedures:
■ The blind introduction of the first trocar should be avoided,- especially when close to a scar -, because the open approach is safer [50; 51].
■ Intraperitoneal pressure should generally be kept to a minimum, especially in patients with cardiac comorbidity, as mentioned above [42].
Some issues in pre- and postoperative therapy have also been tested sufficiently in several randomized clinical trials. From these data it can be concluded, that...
■ ...prophylactic antibiotics are usually dispensable [52-57],
■ ...the general application of intraperitoneal drains is also unneccessary (and if drains are used, they should have not active suction on them) [58-66], and
■ ...routine intravenous infusions after routine LC cause discomfort for the patient without having any relevant clinical benefit [67; 68].

References

(Ref. 1 – 4 relate to high-quality studies, which the original recommendations in 1994 were based on. Ref. 5 – 67 are mainly high-quality studies but also other reports published since then.)

1. Barkun JS, Barkun AN, Sampalis JS, et al. (1992) Randomised controlled trial of laparoscopic versus mini cholecystectomy. The McGill Gallstone Treatment Group. Lancet 340: 1116-1119.

2. Hauer-Jensen M, Kåresen R, Nygaard K, et al. (1993) Prospective randomized study of routine intraoperative cholangiography during open cholecystectomy: long-term follow-up and multivariate analysis of predictors of choledocholithiasis. Surgery 113: 318-323.
3. Kunz R, Orth K, Vogel J, et al. (1992) Laparoskopische Cholezystektomie versus Mini-Lap-Cholezystektomie. Ergebnisse einer prospektiven, randomisierten Studie. Chirurg 63: 291-295.
4. McMahon AJ, Russell IT, Baxter JN, et al. (1994) Laparoscopic versus minilaparotomy cholecystectomy: a randomised trial. Lancet 343: 135-138.
5. Putensen-Himmer G, Putensen C, Lammer H, et al. (1992) Comparison of postoperative respiratory function after laparoscopy or open laparotomy for cholecystectomy. Anesthesiology 77: 675-680.
6. Agnifili A, Ibi I, Guadagni S, et al. (1993) Dolore e stress perioperatori: confronto tra video-laparocolecistectomia e colecistectimia 'open'. G Chir 14: 344-348.
7. Trondsen E, Reiertsen O, Andersen OK, Kjærsgaard P (1993) Laparoscopic and open cholecystectomy. A prospective, randomized study. Eur J Surg 159: 217-221.
8. Schauer PR, Luna J, Ghiatas AA, et al. (1993) Pulmonary function after laparoscopic cholecystectomy. Surgery 114: 389-399.
9. Coelho JC, de Araujo RP, Marchesini JB, Coelho IC, de Araujo LR (1993) Pulmonary function after cholecystectomy performed through Kocher's incision, a mini-incision, and laparoscopy. World J Surg 17: 544-546.
10. Jan YY, Chen MF (1993) [Laparoscopic versus open cholecystectomy: a prospective randomized study]. J Formos Med Assoc 92 Suppl 4: S243-249.
11. Garcia-Caballero M, Vara-Thorbeck C (1993) The evolution of postoperative ileus after laparoscopic cholecystectomy. A comparative study with conventional cholecystectomy and sympathetic blockade treatment. Surg Endosc 7: 416-419.
12. Tate JJ, Lau WY, Leung KL, Li AK (1993) Laparoscopic versus mini-incision cholecystectomy. Lancet 341: 1214-1215.
13. McMahon AJ, O'Dwyer PJ, Cruikshank AM, et al. (1993) Comparison of metabolic responses to laparoscopic and minilaparotomy cholecystectomy. Br J Surg 80: 1255-1258.
14. McMahon AJ, Baxter JN, Kenny G, PJ OD (1993) Ventilatory and blood gas changes during laparoscopic and open cholecystectomy. Br J Surg 80: 1252-1254.
15. McMahon AJ, Russell IT, Ramsay G, et al. (1994) Laparoscopic and minilaparotomy cholecystectomy: a randomized trial comparing postoperative pain and pulmonary function. Surgery 115: 533-539.
16. Byrne J, Timon D, Armstrong C, Horgan PG, Quill DS (1994) A comparion of analgesic requirements and pulmonary function in 'open' versus laparoscopic cholecystectomy. Minimally Invasive Therapy 3: 3-6.
17. Berggren U, Gordh T, Grama D, et al. (1994) Laparoscopic versus open cholecystectomy: hospitalization, sick leave, analgesia and trauma responses. Br J Surg 81: 1362-1365.
18. McMahon AJ, Ross S, Baxter JN, et al. (1995) Symptomatic outcome 1 year after laparoscopic and minilaparotomy cholecystectomy: a randomized trial. Br J Surg 82: 1378-1382.
19. Majeed AW, Troy G, Nicholl JP, et al. (1996) Randomised, prospective, single-blind comparison of laparoscopic versus small-incision cholecystectomy. Lancet 347: 989-994.
20. Squirrell DM, Majeed AW, Troy G, et al. (1998) A randomized, prospective, blinded comparison of postoperative pain, metabolic response, and perceived health after laparoscopic and small incision cholecystectomy. Surgery 123: 485-495.
21. McGinn FP, Miles AJ, Uglow M, et al. (1995) Randomized trial of laparoscopic cholecystectomy and mini-cholecystectomy. Br J Surg 82: 1374-1377.
22. Downs SH, Black NA, Devlin HB (1996) Systematic review of the effectiveness and safety of laparoscopic cholecystectomy. Ann R Coll Surg Engl 78.
23. Paolucci V, Schaeff B, Gutt C, Morawe G, Encke A (1995) Einmal- versus wiederverwendbare Instrumente in der laparoskopischen Chirurgie - eine kontrollierte Untersuchung. Zentralbl Chir 120: 47-52.
24. Leggett PL, Churchman-Winn R, Miller G (2000) Minimizing ports to improve laparoscopic cholecystectomy. Surg Endosc 14: 32-36.

25. Bresadola F, Pasqualucci A, Donini A, et al. (1999) Elective transumbilical compared with standard laparoscopic cholecystectomy. Eur J Surg 165: 29-34.
26. Tsimoyiannis EC, Jabarin M, Glantzounis G, et al. (1998) Laparoscopic cholecystectomy using ultrasonically activated coagulating shears. Surg Laparosc Endosc 8: 421-424.
27. Hanna GB, Shimi SM, Cuschieri A (1998) Randomised study of influence of two-dimensional versus three-dimensional imaging on performance of laparoscopic cholecystectomy. Lancet 351: 248-251.
28. Wallace DH, Serpell MG, Baxter JN, O'Dwyer PJ (1997) Randomized trial of different insufflation pressures for laparoscopic cholecystectomy. Br J Surg 84: 455-458.
29. Lindgren L, Koivusalo AM, Kellokumpu I (1995) Conventional pneumoperitoneum compared with abdominal wall lift for laparoscopic cholecystectomy. Br J Anaesth 75: 567-572.
30. Kitano S, Iso Y, Tomikawa M, Moriyama M, Sugimachi K (1993) A prospective randomized trial comparing pneumoperitoneum and U-shaped retractor elevation for laparoscopic cholecystectomy. Surg Endosc 7: 311-314.
31. Mouton WG, Bessell JR, Millard SH, Baxter PS, Maddern GJ (1999) A randomized controlled trial assessing the benefit of humidified insufflation gas during laparoscopic surgery. Surg Endosc 13: 106-108.
32. Puttick MI, Scott-Coombes DM, Dye J, et al. (1999) Comparison of immunologic and physiologic effects of CO_2 pneumoperitoneum at room and body temperatures. Surg Endosc 13: 572-575.
33. Slim K, Bousquet J, Kwiatkowski F, et al. (1999) Effect of CO_2 gas warming on pain after laparoscopic surgery: a randomized double-blind controlled trial. Surg Endosc 13: 1110-1114.
34. Redmond HP, Watson RW, Houghton T, et al. (1994) Immune function in patients undergoing open vs laparoscopic cholecystectomy. Arch Surg 129: 1240-1246.
35. Dauleh MI, Rahman S, Townell NH (1995) Open versus laparoscopic cholecystectomy: a comparison of postoperative temperature. J R Coll Surg Edinb 40: 116-118.
36. Karayiannakis AJ, Makri GG, Mantzioka A, Karousos D, Karatzas G (1996) Postoperative pulmonary function after laparoscopic and open cholecystectomy. Br J Anaesth 77: 448-452.
37. Chumillas MS, Ponce JL, Delgado F, Viciano V (1998) Pulmonary function and complications after laparoscopic cholecystectomy. Eur J Surg 164: 433-437.
38. Prisco D, De Gaudio AR, Carla R, et al. (2000) Videolaparoscopic cholecystectomy induces a hemostasis activation of lower grade than does open surgery. Surg Endosc 14: 170-174.
39. Ortega AE, Peters JH, Incarbone R, et al. (1996) A prospective randomized comparison of the metabolic and stress hormonal responses of laparoscopic and open cholecystectomy. J Am Coll Surg 183: 249-256.
40. Karayiannakis AJ, Makri GG, Mantzioka A, Karousos D, Karatzas G (1997) Systemic stress response after laparoscopic or open cholecystectomy: a randomized trial. Br J Surg 84: 467-471.
41. Wills VL, Hunt DR (2000) Pain after laparoscopic cholecystectomy. Br J Surg 87: 273-284.
42. Dexter SP, Vucevic M, Gibson J, McMahon MJ (1999) Hemodynamic consequences of high- and low-pressure capnoperitoneum during laparoscopic cholecystectomy. Surg Endosc 13: 376-381.
43. Morino M, Giraudo G, Festa V (1998) Alterations in hepatic function during laparoscopic surgery. An experimental clinical study. Surg Endosc 12: 968-972.
44. Vezakis A, Davides D, Gibson JS, et al. (1999) Randomized comparison between low-pressure laparoscopic cholecystectomy and gasless laparoscopic cholecystectomy. Surg Endosc 13: 890-893.
45. McArthur P, Cuschieri A, Sells RA, Shields R (1975) Controlled clinical trial comparing early with interval cholecystectomy for acute cholecystitis. Br J Surg 62: 850-852.
46. Kiviluoto T, Siren J, Luukkonen P, Kivilaakso E (1998) Randomised trial of laparoscopic versus open cholecystectomy for acute and gangrenous cholecystitis. Lancet 351: 321-325.
47. Cohen MM, Young W, Theriault ME, Hernandez R (1996) Has laparoscopic cholecystectomy changed patterns of practice and patient outcome in Ontario? CMAJ 154: 491-500.

48. Russell JC, Walsh SJ, Mattie AS, Lynch JT (1996) Bile duct injuries, 1989-1993. A statewide experience. Connecticut Laparoscopic Cholecystectomy Registry. Arch Surg 131: 382-388.
49. Fletcher DR, Hobbs MS, Tan P, et al. (1999) Complications of cholecystectomy: risks of the laparoscopic approach and protective effects of operative cholangiography: a population-based study. Ann Surg 229: 449-457.
50. Cogliandolo A, Manganaro T, Saitta FP, Micali B (1998) Blind versus open approach to laparoscopic cholecystectomy: a randomized study. Surg Laparosc Endosc 8: 353-355.
51. Ostrzenski A (1999) Randomized, prospective, single-blind trial of a new parallel technique of Veress pneumoperitoneum needle insertion versus the conventional closed method. Fertil Steril 71: 578-581.
52. Illig KA, Schmidt E, Cavanaugh J, Krusch D, Sax HC (1997) Are prophylactic antibiotics required for elective laparoscopic cholecystectomy? J Am Coll Surg 184: 353-356.
53. Lewis RT, Weigand FM, Mamazza J, Lloyd-Smith W, Tataryn D (1995) Should antibiotic prophylaxis be used routinely in clean surgical procedures: a tentative yes. Surgery 118: 742-747.
54. Higgins A, London J, Charland S, et al. (1999) Prophylactic antibiotics for elective laparoscopic cholecystectomy: are they necessary? Arch Surg 134: 611-614.
55. Dobay KJ, Freier DT, Albear P (1999) The absent role of prophylactic antibiotics in low-risk patients undergoing laparoscopic cholecystectomy. Am Surg 65: 226-228.
56. Tocchi A, Lepre L, Costa G, et al. (2000) The need for antibiotic prophylaxis in elective laparoscopic cholecystectomy: a prospective randomized study. Arch Surg 135: 67-70.
57. Paraskevopoulos JA, Samoilis S, Kostopoulos O, et al. (2000) Systemic antibiotic prophylaxis in laparoscopic cholecystectomy: a necessity or an obsolete policy? [abstract]. Surg Endosc 14(Suppl.1): S139.
58. Cogliandolo A, Manganaro T, Aloisi G, Pidotti RR, Micali B (1995) Usefulness of drainage after laparoscopic cholecystectomy. A randomized study. Endosurgery 3: 110-112.
59. Hawasli A, Brown E (1994) The effect of drains in laparoscopic cholecystectomy. J Laparoendosc Surg 4: 393-398.
60. Saad AM, el Hassan AM (1993) Cholecystectomy with and without drainage: a prospective randomised study. East Afr Med J 70: 499-501.
61. Kapoor VK, Ibrarullah M, Baijal SS, et al. (1993) Cholecystectomy and drainage: ultrasonographic and radioisotopic evaluation. World J Surg 17: 101-104.
62. al-Arfaj AL, Shahab K, al-Ghassab G, et al. (1992) Drainage after cholecystectomy. A prospective randomized clinical trial. Int Surg 77: 274-276.
63. Kriplani AK, Sawhney S, Kumar S, Kapur BM (1992) Influence of intraperitoneal drainage after cholecystectomy; a prospective ultrasonographic study. Trop Gastroenterol 13: 146-151.
64. Förster R, Schnabel M, Krahl M, Lindlar R, Rothmund M (1992) Routinedrainage nach unkomplizierter, elektiver Cholecystektomie? Eine prospektive, randomisierte Studie. Chirurg 63: 558-562.
65. Monson JRT, Guillou PJ, Keane FBV, Tanner WA, Brennan TG (1991) Cholecystectomy is safer without drainage: the results of a prospective, randomized clinical trial. Surgery 109: 740-746.
66. Jorgensen JO, Gillies RB, Hunt DR, Caplehorn JR, Lumley T (1995) A simple and effective way to reduce postoperative pain after laparoscopic cholecystectomy. Aust N Z J Surg 65: 466-469.
67. Robertson GS, Bundred NJ, Bullen BR, Moshakis V (1992) A drip is unnecessary after cholecystectomy. J R Coll Surg Edinb 37: 244-246.
68. Salim AS (1991) Duration of intravenous fluid replacement after abdominal surgery: a prospective randomised study. Ann R Coll Surg Engl 73: 119-123.

Laparoscopic antireflux surgery for gastroesophageal reflux disease (GERD)

E.A.E.S. Consensus Development Conference (1997)[1,2] with updating comments (2000)

Conference organizers (1996):

E. Eypasch, Surgical Clinic Merheim, 2nd Department of Surgery, University of Cologne (Germany);
E. Neugebauer, Biochemical and Experimental Division, 2nd Department of Surgery, University of Cologne (Germany);
F. Fischer, Surgical Clinic Merheim, 2nd Department of Surgery, University of Cologne (Germany);
H. Troidl, Surgical Clinic Merheim, 2nd Department of Surgery, University of Cologne (Germany);

Expert Panel (1996):

A. L. Blum, Division de Gastro-Entérologie, Centre Hospitalier, Universitaire Vaudois (CHUV) Lausanne (Switzerland);
D. Collet, Department of Surgery, University of Bordeaux (France);
A. Cuschieri, Department of Surgery, Ninewells Hospital & Medical School, University of Dundee, Dundee, Scotland (U.K.);
B. Dallemagne, Department of Surgery, Saint Joseph Hospital, Liège (Belgium);
H. Feussner, Chirurgische Klinik u. Poliklinik rechts der Isar, Universität München, München (Germany);
K.-H. Fuchs; Chirurgische Universitätsklinik und Poliklinik Würzburg, Universität Würzburg, Würzburg (Germany);

---

1) Held at the 4th International Congress of the European Association for Endoscopic Surgery (E.A.E.S.), Trondheim, Norway, 21-24 June, 1996
2) The original conference is published in Surg Endosc (1997) 11: 413-426.

H. GLISE, Department of Surgery, Norra Älvsborgs Länssjukhus, Trollhättan (Sweden);

C. K. KUM, Department of Surgery, National University Hospital, Singapore (Singapore);

T. LERUT, Department of Thoracic Surgery, University Hospital Leuven, Leuven (Belgium);

L. LUNDELL, Department of Surgery, Sahlgren's Hospital, University of Göteborg, Göteborg (Sweden);

H. E. MYRVOLD, Department of Surgery, Regionsykehuset, University of Trondheim, Trondheim (Norway);

A. PERACCHIA, Department of Surgery, University of Milan, School of Medicine, Milan (Italy);

H. PETERSEN, Department of Medicine, Regionsykehuset, University of Trondheim, Trondheim (Norway);

J. J. B. VAN LANSCHOT, Department of Surgery, Academisch Ziekenhuis, University of Amsterdam, Amsterdam (Netherlands)

Updating comments (2000):

E. EYPASCH, Department of Surgery, Malteser Krankenhaus St.Hildegardis, Köln-Lindenthal (Germany)

Consensus statements (1996)

Question 1. What are the epidemiologic facts in GERD?

In western countries, gastroesophageal reflux has a high prevalence and, in the USA and Europe in up to 44% of the adult population describe symptoms characteristic for GERD. Troublesome symptoms characteristic for GERD occur in 10-15% with equal frequency in men and women. Men, however, seem to develop reflux esophagitis and complications of esophagitis more frequently than women. Data from the literature indicate that 10-50% of these subjects will need long-term treatment of some kind for their symptoms and/or esophagitis.

The panelists agreed that the natural history of the disease varies in a wide spectrum between very benign and harmless reflux to a disabling stage of the disease with severe symptoms and endoscopic alterations. There are no good long-term data indicating how the natural history of the disease changes from one stage to the other and when and how complications (esophagitis, stricture, etc.) develop.

Further topics of considerable debate which could not be resolved within this conference are:
- the cause of the increasing prevalence of esophagitis
- the cause of the increasing prevalence of Barrett's esophagus and adenocarcinoma
- the discrepancy between clinically and anatomically determined prevalence of Barrett's esophagus
- the problem of ultra-short Barrett's esophagus and its meaning
- the relationship between *Helicobacter pylori* infection and reflux esophagitis
- gastroesophageal reflux without esophagitis and abnormal sensitivity of the esophagus to acid, and
- the role of so-called alkaline reflux which is currently difficult to measure objectively.

Question 2. What is the current pathophysiological concept of GERD?

GERD is a multifactorial process in which esophageal and gastric changes are involved. Major causes involved in the pathophysiology are incompetence of the lower esophageal sphincter expressed as low sphincter length and pressure and frequent transient lower esophageal sphincter relaxations, insufficient esophageal peristalsis, altered esophageal mucosal resistance, delayed gastric emptying, and antroduodenal motility disorders with pathologic duodeno-gastro-esophageal reflux.

Several factors can play an aggravating role: stress, posture, obesity, pregnancy, dietary factors (e.g. fat, chocolate, caffeine, fruit juice, peppermint, alcohol, spicy food) and drugs (e.g. calcium antagonists, anticholinergics, theophylline, ß-blockers, dihydropridine). All these factors might influence the pressure gradient from the abdomen to the chest either by decreasing the lower esophageal sphincter or by increasing abdominal pressure.

Further parts of the physiological mosaic that might contribute to gastroesophageal reflux are the circadian rhythm of sphincter pressure, gastric and salivary secretion, esophageal clearance mechanisms as well as hiatal hernia and *Helicobacter pylori* infection.

Question 3. Which is a useful definition of the disease?

A universally agreed scientific classification of GERD is not yet available. A current model of gastroesophageal reflux disease is an excessive exposure of the mucosa to of gastric contents (amount and composition) causing symptoms accompanied and/or caused by different pathophysiological phenomena (sphincter pressure, peristalsis) leading to morphological changes (esophagitis, cell infiltration).

This implies an abnormal exposure to acid and/or other gastric contents like bile, duodenal and pancreatic juice in cases of a combined duodeno-gastroesophageal reflux.

The classification of GERD is frequently synonymously used with the classification of esophagitis, even though there is a lot of evidence that only 60% of patients with reflux disease sustain damage of their mucosa. The MUSE or Savary esophagitis classification are currently used for the staging of the damage, but they are poor for the staging of the disease.

The modified AFP-Score (Anatomy-Function-Pathology) is an attempt to incorporate the presence of hiatus hernia, reflux, macroscopic and morphologic damage in the classification. However, this classification lacks symptomatology and should be linked to a scoring system for symptoms or quality of life; both scoring systems which are extremely important for staging of the disease and for the indication for treatment.

Question 4. What establishes the diagnosis of the disease?

A large variety of different symptoms is described in the context of gastroesophageal reflux disease, such as dysphagia, pharyngeal pain, hoarseness, nausea, belching, epigastric pain, retrosternal pain, acid and food regurgitation, retrosternal burning, heartburn, retrosternal pressure and coughing. The characteristic symptoms are heartburn (retrosternal burning), regurgitation, pain and coughing. Symptoms are usually related to posture and eating habits.

In addition, typical reflux patients may have symptoms which are not located in the region of the esophagus. Patients with heartburn may or may not have pathological reflux. They may belong to the group of patients with reflux -type "non ulcer dyspepsia" or other functional disorders.

The diagnostic tests that are needed must follow a certain algorithm. After the history and physical examination of the patients, an upper gastrointestinal endoscopy is performed. A biopsy is taken if any abnormalities (stenosis, strictures, Barrett`s etc.) are found.

If no morphologic evidence can be detected, only functional studies, e.g. measuring the acid exposure in the esophageal lumen by 24h esophageal pH monitoring, are helpful and indicated to detect excessive reflux. It is of vital importance that the pH-electrode is accurately positioned in relation to the lower esophageal sphincter (LES). Manometry is the only objective way of assessing the location of the LES. Ordinary esophageal radiologic studies (barium swallow) are considered another mandatory basic imaging study.

In the next level of investigations there are a number of tests to look for the cause of pathologic reflux either by esophageal manometry as a basic investigation for this purpose to assess lower esophageal sphincter and esophageal body function. Videoesophagography or esophageal emptying scintigraphy may also be helpful.

Table 1: Diagnostic Test Ranking Order for GERD

Basic diagnostic tests	Physiologic/ pathologic Criteria
Endoscopy + Histology	Savary-Miller classification (I, II, II, IV,V) MUSE classification: Metaplasia – Ulcer – Stricture - Erosions
Radiology	Barium swallow
24-h esophageal pH monitoring	percentage time below pH 4 DeMeester score
Stationary esophageal manometry*	Lower esophageal sphincter: - overall length, - intraabdominal length, - pressure (transient LES relaxations) esophageal body disorders weak peristalsis
Optional tests	
24h gastric pH monitoring	persistent gastric acidity excessive duodenogastric reflux
Gastric emptying scintigraphy	Delayed gastric emptying
Photo-optic bilirubin assessment	Esophageal bile exposure Gastric bile exposure

Optional gastric function studies are 24h gastric pH monitoring, photo-optic bilirubin assessment to assess duodenogastroesophageal reflux, gastric emptying scintigraphy or antroduodenal manometry. Currently these gastric function studies are of scientific interest but they do not yet play a role in overall clinical patient management, apart from selected patients. The diagnostic test ranking order is displayed in **Table 1**.

Table 2: Literature evidence on antireflux operations and medical treatment

Issue	Level III studies (i.e. randomised controlled trials)
Antireflux surgery	[1-4]
Medical treatment	[5-33]

Question 5. What is the indication for treatment?

Pivotal criteria for the indication to medical treatment in gastroesophageal reflux disease are the patient's symptoms, reduced quality of life, and the general condition of the patient. When symptoms persist or recur after medication, endoscopy is strongly indicated.

Mucosal damage (esophagitis) indicates a strong need for medical treatment. If the symptoms persist, partially persist, or recur after stopping medication, there is a good indication for doing functional studies. Gastrointestinal endoscopy, already mentioned as the basic imaging examination in GERD should be performed in context with the functional studies.

Indication for surgery is again centrally based on the patient's symptoms, the duration of the symptoms and the damage that is present. Even after successful medical acid suppression the patient can have persistent or recurrent symptoms of epigastric pain and retrosternal pressure as well as food regurgitation due to the incompetent cardia, insufficient peristalsis, and/or a large hiatal hernia.

With respect to indication, one important factor in the patient's general condition is age. On the one hand, age plays a role in risk stratification when the individual risk of an operation is estimated together with the co-morbidity of the patient. On the other hand, age is an economic factor with to respect ot the break-even point between medical and surgical therapy.

Concerning the indication for surgery, a differentiation in the symptoms between heartburn and regurgitation is considered important. (Medical treatment appears to be more effective for heartburn than for regurgitation.)

Therefore the indication of surgery is based on the following facts:

■ Noncompliance of the patient with ongoing effective medical treatment. Reasons for noncompliance are preference, refusal, reduced quality of life, or drug dependency and drug side effects.

■ Persistent or recurrent esophagitis in spite of currently optimal medical treatment and in association with symptoms.

■ Complications of the disease (stenoses, ulcers and Barrett's esophagus) have a minor influence on the indication. Neither medical nor surgical treatment have been shown to alter the extent of Barrett's epithelium.

Therefore mainly symptoms and their relation to ongoing medical treatment play the major role for the indication for surgery. However, antireflux surgery may reduce the need for subsequent endoscopic dilatations. The participants pointed out that patients with symptoms completely resistent to antisecretory treatment with H2-blockers or proton pump inhibitors are bad candidates for surgery. In these individuals other diseases have to be investigated carefully. On the contrary, good candidates for surgery should have a good response to antisecretory drugs. Thus, compliance and preference determine which treatment is chosen (conservative or operative).

Question 6. What are the essentials of laparoscopic surgical treatment?

The goal of surgical treatment for GERD is to relieve the symptoms and to prevent progression and complications of the disease by the creation of a new anatomical high-pressure zone. This must be achieved without dysphagia, which can occur when the outflow resistance of the reconstructed GE junction exceeds the peristaltic power of the body of the oesophagus. Achievement of this goal requires an understanding of the natural history of GERD, the status of patient's esophageal function and a selection of the appropriate antireflux procedure.

Since the newly created structure is only a substitute for the lower esophageal sphincter, it is a matter of discussion to what extent it can show physiological reactions (normal resting pressure, reaction to pharmacological stimuli, appropriate relaxations during deglutition, etc.). There is no agreement on how surgical procedures work and restore the gastroesophageal reflux barrier.

With respect to the details of the laparoscopic surgical procedures, the following degree of consensus was attained by the panel (11 present participants) (yes/no):

1. Is there a need for mobilisation of the gastric fundus by dividing the short gastric vessels? (7/4)

2. Is there a need for dissection of the crura? (11/0)

3. Is there a need for identification of the vagal trunks? (7/4)

4. Is there a need for removal of the esophageal fat pad? (2/9)

5. Is there a need for closure of the crura posteriorly? (11/0)

6. Should non-absorbable sutures be used (crura, wrap) (11/0)

7. Should a large bougie (40-60 French) used for calibration (5/6)

8. Should objective assessment be performed (e.g. calibration by a bougie, others) for tightness of the hiatus and tightness of the wrap? (9/0 resp. 9/2)

9. If there is normal peristalsis, should one routinely use a 360° short floppy fundoplication wrap, a partial fundoplication wrap, or a short wrap (< 2,5 cm length)? (8/2/1)

10. In cases of weak peristalsis, should there "tailored approach" (total or partial wrap)? (5/6)

Question 7. Which are the important endpoints of treatment whether medical or surgical?

The important endpoints for the success of conservative/medical as well as surgical therapy must be the mosaic of different criteria, since neither clinical symptoms, functional criteria nor the daily activity and quality of life assessment can be used solely to assess the therapeutic result in this multifactorial disease process.

Patients show a great variety in demonstrating and expressing the severity of clinical symptoms and, therefore, they alone are not a reliable guide. Functional criteria can be assessed objectively, but may not be used in the decision making process without looking at the stage of mucosal damage or morphological abnormalities (hiatus hernia, slipped wrap; AFP-Score).

Complete evaluation includes assessment of symptoms, daily activity and quality of life, ideally in every single patient. The earliest point to collect functional data after the operation is 6 months. The reasonable time of assessment in the post-surgical follow-up phase is probably 1 year followed by 2 year intervals. Economic assessment is considered to be a significant endpoint and is dealt with in a later section.

There is no evidence that laparoscopic surgery should be any better than conventional surgery. If laparoscopic surgery is correctly performed, apart from the problems of abdominal wall complications like hernia, infection and wound rupture, there should be no difference in outcome as compared to the standard obtained in open surgery. Laparoscopic surgery, however, has the potential to reduce post-operative pain and limitations of daily activity.

Question 8. What is failure of treatment?

In gastroesophageal reflux disease, life-long medication is needed in many patients, because the disease persists and the acid reduction can take away the symptoms during the time the medication is taken. Therefore the disease is treated by reducing the acid and not by treating or correcting the causes of the disease. This latter argument can be used by the surgeons since they mechanically restore the sphincter area and, therefore, correct the most frequent defect associated with the disease.

In surgery, failure of a treatment is defined as the persistence or recurrence of symptoms and/or objective pathologic findings once the treatment phase is finished. In GERD, a definite failure is present, when symptoms which are severe enough to require at least intermittent therapy (heartburn, regurgitation) recur after treatment or when other serious problems ("slipped Nissen", severe gas bloat syndrome, dumping syndrome etc.) arise and when functional studies document that symptoms are due to this problem. Recurrence can occur with or without esophageal damage (esophagitis). Professor Blum (Lausanne) suggested that further long-term outcome studies of medical and surgical treatment are needed.

Quality of life measurements are able to differentiate whether and to what extent recurrent symptoms are really impairing the patient' s quality of life.

It was agreed upon that a distinction is necessary between the two types of failures of the operation: "the unhappy 5-10%" (i.e. slipped Nissen, etc.) and the 10-40% of individuals who become only aware of their dyspeptic symptoms postoperatively while the reflux related symptoms are treated. Dyspeptic symptoms occur in the normal population in 20-40%). Some of the "post-fundoplication symptoms" are present already before the operation and are due to the dyspeptic symptomatology associated with GERD.

Patients with failures should be worked up with the available diagnostic tests to detect the underlying cause of the failure. If there is mild recurrent reflux, it usually can be treated by medication, as long as the patient is satisfied with this solution and his/her quality of life is good. In the case of severe symptomatic recurrent reflux or other complications and if endoscopy shows visible esophagitis, the indication for refundoplication after a thorough diagnostic work-up must be established. Surgeons very experienced in pathophysiology, diagnosis and the surgical technique of the disease should perform these redo operations. Expert management of patients undergoing redo surgery for a benign condition is of extreme importance.

Question 9. What are the issues in an economic evaluation?

With respect to a complete economic evaluation the panelists refer to the available literature. Cost, cost minimisation and cost effectiveness analyses of gastroesophageal reflux disease must take into account the costs of the following issues (list incomplete): Medications, office visits, routine endoscopies, frequency of sick leaves at work, frequency of restricted family or hobby activity at home, assessment of job performance and restrictions due to the disease, diagnostic work-up including functional studies and specialised investigations, surgical intervention, treatment of surgical complications, treatment of complications of maintenance medical therapy, such as emergency hospital admissions, e.g. swallowing discomfort, bolus entrapment in peptic stenoses, perspective of the analysis (patient, hospital, society), and health care system (socialized, private). A special issue is the so-called break-even-point between medical and surgical treatment (duration and cost of medical treatment versus laparoscopic antireflux treatment.

Ultimately, the results of medical or surgical treatment, especially with respect to age of the patient should be translated into quality adjusted life years (QALYs) to differentiate which treatment is better for what age, co-morbidity and stage of disease.

Question 10a. What stage of technological development are endoscopic antireflux operations at (in June 1996)?

Technical performance and applicability have been demonstrated by several authors as early as 1992/1993. The results on safety, complications, morbidity and mortality data depend on the learning phase (> 50 cases) of the operations. The complication, reoperation, and conversion rates are higher in the first 20 cases of an individual surgeon. It is strongly advocated that experienced supervision is sought by surgeons beginning laparoscopic fundoplication during their first 20 procedures. Data on efficacy (benefit for the patient) demonstrated in centres of excellence were based on type II studies. The benefit for the surgeon in terms of elegance, ease, and speed of the procedure is not yet clear cut. The operation time is the same or longer, the technique is harder initially,- however, the view of the operating field is better. The effectiveness data are still insufficient, long-term results are missing, and the results reported come mainly from interested centres and multicenter studies. It is important to audit continually the results of antireflux operations, especially because different techniques are used. The economic evaluation of laparoscopic antireflux surgery is still premature (few data from small studies only). Future studies are recommended in different health care systems, assessing the relative economic advantages of laparoscopic antireflux surgery in comparison to the available and paid medical treatment.

A major issue of ethical concern is the altered indication for surgery. A change of indication might produce more cost and harm in inappropriately selected patients. Laparoscopic antireflux surgery should be recommended in centres with sufficient experience and an adequate number of individuals with the disease. Randomized controlled studies are recommended to compare medical vs laparoscopic surgical treatment and partial vs total fundoplication wraps.

Question 10b. What is the current status of laparoscopic antireflux surgery vs open conventional procedures in terms of feasibility and efficacy parameters?

The evaluation is mainly based on type I and type II studies (see list of references). The results show that safety is comparable and rather favourable compared to the open technique. The incidence for complications, morbidity and mortality is similar to the open technique once the learning phase has been surpassed. In terms of efficacy significant advantages of the endoscopic antireflux operations are: less postoperative pain, shorter hospital stay and earlier return to normal activities and work.

In general, laparoscopic antireflux surgery has advantages over open conventional procedures if performed by trained surgeons. Laparoscopic antireflux surgery has the potential to improve reflux treatment provided that appropriate diagnostic facilities for functional esophageal studies and adequately trained and dedicated surgeons are available.

Updating comments (2000)

Background – The original CDC on reflux disease

The consensus statements from 1996 addressed 11 questions: Nine questions were on more general issues of GERD and two described laparoscopic antireflux surgery according to the criteria of technology assessment. The consensus statements 1 to 5 dealt with epidemiology, pathophysiology, definition, diagnosis of the disease as well as indication for treatment, especially surgical intervention. In other words, these statements covered some general aspects of gastroesophageal reflux disease which should be covered according to the current state of knowledge.

The best available evidence from the literature was collected using a strategy similar to evidence-based medicine. The 13 selected experts including several highly respected medical gastroenterologists were physically present discussing for almost 12 hours. Nevertheless, the consensus statements presented to the surgical public at that time were looked upon as boring, not original enough and too weak. A highlight and a novelty, however, was the second section of consensus statement 5 which pointed out that indication for surgery was based on non-compliance of the patient with ongoing medical treatment due to personal preference, refusal to take drugs, reduced quality of life, drug dependence and side effects. For the first time this clearly pointed out the preference of a patient to choose between the 2 treatment option: medical or surgical.

Questions 7 to 9 dealt with the endpoints of treatment, treatment failure, and special issues on economic evaluation,– again not fascinating for the public. Economic evaluation of antireflux surgery was a white spot on the landmap at that time.

Needless to say, that the surgical interest focused on technical principles and details of the laparoscopic operation itself. Within consensus statement 6, technical details were broken down in ten aspects each of which was put up to a vote by the experts. The results of the vote are shown above (Question 6). While some surgical steps of the operation were agreed upon unanimously (dissection of crura, non-absorbable sutures) others caused considerable and constant dissent: i.e. modification of the wrap and mobilization of the gastric fundus.

In terms of technology assessment, laparoscopic antireflux surgery was considered better with respect to intraoperative spleen and vessel injuries, wound infections, abdominal wall hernias, postoperative pain, recovery and activities, hospital stay and cosmesis. In most of the other items there was no difference or a slight disadvantage found for i.e. emphysema and operative time. With a consensus of 60 %, laparoscopic surgery was assessed as superior. The drawback, caveat or the drop of vermouth in the wine, however, is that this consensus was based on studies with a degree of evidence I to II only. This reflected a considerable lack of randomized controlled trials to support the consensus.

In conclusion – if a single author is allowed to conclude – the consensus of 1996 was evident, however based on weak data, revealing a lack of information, attractivenes and originality. A French surgeon commented that the document stimulated your appetite but left you still hungry.

Methods of literature search

To retrieve all relevant literature concerning the consensus questions, an extensive literature search was undertaken. Key words for the literature search were "gastroesophageal reflux disease, esophagitis, surgery, and consensus". The search was limited to Medline for the 24-month period from the middle of 1997 to 1999.

The whole amount of publications came to 714 articles resulting in about 1 publication per day (714 per 730 days). The papers were screened for review articles, randomized clinical trials and reports of other consecutive consensus conferences about reflux disease. All the available randomized trials were studied in detail and their reference lists was analysed. Interestingly 5 of the 6 randomized clinical trials focus on the technical details of the operation as shown in Table 1 where they can be compared to the original consensus statements.

Results of recent randomized controlled trials

In a prospective double-blind randomized trial, Watson and Jamieson addressed the topic of performing the laparoscopic Nissen procedure with or without division of the short gastric vessels [34]. One hundred and two patients were entered into the trial. The endpoint of the study were dysphagia, heartburn, and patient satisfaction, each one assessed on a standardized clinical grading system 1, 3 and 6 months after surgery. Although the operating time was increased by 40 minutes, the authors did not detect a benefit in clinical outcome due to a division of the short gastric vessels.

The same issue of mobilization of the gastric fundus (by dividing the short gastric vessels) –although still in open surgery - was addressed by the randomized study of Luostarinen and Isolauri [35]. Fifty consecutive patients were randomized to open conventional Nissen-Rosetti fundopliaction with or without total fundic mobilization. Fundic mobilization did not show any advantage regarding postoperative adverse effects, however, it was associated with a higher rate of recurrent hiatal hernia in 9 out of 26 patients with mobilization (35 %!). Thus, another study failed to show a benefit of fundic mobilization.

The study by Laws dealt with the issue of performing a complete or a partial fundoplication wrap [36]. In 42 patients of whom 23 were assigned to a total (Nissen), and 16 to a partial (Toupet) wrap, the investigators used the Visick classification to grade the results. At follow-up visits, Visick scores were I in 13, II in 8 and III in 2 patients after the complete wrap and I in 12 and II in 3 individuals after the partial wrap. The authors conclude that there is no clear advantage of one wrap over the other. Although the type of the study can lead to results of evidence grade III, the low number of patients and the crude and not-validated Visick score imply that the results should be interpreted with some caution.

Also the recent randomized trial by Watson studied the wrap modifications comparing a laparoscopic Nissen fundoplication in 53 patients to an anterior partial reconstruction in 54 individuals [37]. Partial anterior fundoplication resulted in lower resting and residual pressures of the lower sphincter accompanied by a faster oesophageal emptying. At 6 months, the patients with a partial fundoplication had significantly less dysphagia and were more likely satisfied with the operation. The durability of the operation, however, remains a matter of interest for the further follow-up of this trial.

Finally, in a third study, the wrap problem was addressed with special interest to the concept of "tailoring antireflux surgery" to the individual physiological functional of the oesophagus [38]. According to this hypothesis, some researchers recommend a partial "weaker" wrap for individuals with a weaker peristalsis of the oesophageal body. In the study by Rydberg and Lundell irrespective of pre-existing motility disturbances, 106 patients were randomized to either total Nissen-Rosetti or posterior partial Toupet fundoplication [38]. The endpoints of the study were postoperative dysphagia and other oesophageal symptoms. The authors were unable to prove the hypothesis and failed to demonstrate a relation between preoperative manometric findings and postoperative symptoms. The latter was even true for the subgroup of patients with defined pre-existing oesophageal motor abnormalities.

A sixth randomized study focussed on health economic issues. The Finnish authors randomized 42 patients to either laparoscopic or open Nissen Fundoplication [39]. Quality of life (Gastrointestinal Quality of Life Index - GIQLI) and costs were the endpoints of the trial. Although hospital costs were comparable, total costs for laparoscopic surgery only came to half of those for open surgery (7,506 $ versus 13,118 $). While quality of life and overall patient satisfaction were comparable, convalescence with return to work and normal activities was faster after endoscopic surgery.

Conclusion

The discussion of these studies and their integration into a consensus document cannot be done by a single author and would again require detailed debate among the experts. Nevertheless, it can be argued that the degree of evidence for already known and described statements in the consensus document has risen from level II to level III in some aspects, i.e. technical details of the operation. Further examples for the consolidation of the strength of evidence towards grade II are pain, recovery, hospital stay, and costs as variables of technology assessment. They are described in numerous of the above mentioned 714 articles.

In the described literature search also several other consensus conferences on GERD were identified [40-43]. A detailed comparison of the recommendations or a meta-analysis of the randomised studies would go far beyond the scope of this article.

References

(Ref. 1 – 33 relate to high-quality studies, which the original recommendations in 1994 were based on. Ref. 34 – 43 are mainly high-quality studies but also other reports published since then.)

1. Ortiz A, Martinez de Haro LF, Parrilla P, et al. (1996) Conservative treatment versus antireflux surgery in Barrett's oesophagus: long-term results of a prospective study. Br J Surg 83: 274-278.
2. Laine S, Rantala A, Gullichsen R, Ovaska J (1997) Laparoscopic vs conventional Nissen fundoplication. A prospective randomized study. Surg Endosc 11: 441-444.
3. Spechler SJP (1992) Comparison of medical and surgical therapy for complicated gastroesophageal reflux disease in veterans. The Department of Veterans Affairs Gastroesophageal Reflux Disease Study Group. N Engl J Med 326: 786-792.
4. Watson DI, Jamieson GG, Pike GK, et al. (1999) Prospective randomized double-blind trial between laparoscopic Nissen fundoplication and anterior partial fundoplication. Br J Surg 86: 123-130.
5. Arvanitakis C, Nikopoulos A, Theoharidis A, et al. (1993) Cisapride and ranitidine in the treatment of gastro-oesophageal reflux disease--a comparative randomized double-blind trial. Aliment Pharmacol Ther 7: 635-641.
6. Behar J, Sheahan DG, Biancani P, Spiro HM, Storer EH (1975) Medical and surgical management of reflux esophagitis. A 38-month report of a prospective clinical trial. N Engl J Med 293: 263-268.
7. Blum AL, Adami B, Bouzo MH, et al. (1993) Effect of cisapride on relapse of esophagitis. A multinational, placebo-controlled trial in patients healed with an antisecretory drug. The Italian Eurocis Trialists. Dig Dis Sci 38: 551-560.
8. Chopra BK, Kazal HL, Mittal PK, Sibia SS (1992) A comparison of the clinical efficacy of ranitidine and sucralfate in reflux oesophagitis. J Assoc Physicians India 40: 162-163.
9. Dakkak M, Jones BP, Scott MG, Tooley PJ, Bennett JR (1994) Comparing the efficacy of cisapride and ranitidine in oesophagitis: a double-blind, parallel group study in general practice. Br J Clin Pract 48: 10-14.

10. Dent J, Yeomans ND, Mackinnon M, et al. (1994) Omeprazole v ranitidine for prevention of relapse in reflux oesophagitis. A controlled double blind trial of their efficacy and safety. Gut 35: 590-598.

11. Hallerback B, Unge P, Carling L, et al. (1994) Omeprazole or ranitidine in long-term treatment of reflux esophagitis. The Scandinavian Clinics for United Research Group. Gastroenterology 107: 1305-1311.

12. Hatlebakk JG, Berstad A, Carling L, et al. (1993) Lansoprazole versus omeprazole in short-term treatment of reflux oesophagitis. Results of a Scandinavian multicentre trial. Scand J Gastroenterol 28: 224-228.

13. Havelund T, Laursen LS, Skoubo-Kristensen E, et al. (1988) Omeprazole and ranitidine in treatment of reflux oesophagitis: double blind comparative trial. Br Med J 296: 89-92.

14. Hetzel DJ (1992) Controlled clinical trials of omeprazole in the long-term management of reflux disease. Digestion 51 Suppl 1: 35-42.

15. Hetzel DJ, Dent J, Reed WD, et al. (1988) Healing and relapse of severe peptic esophagitis after treatment with omeprazole. Gastroenterology 95: 903-912.

16. Johansson KE, Tibbling L (1986) Maintenance treatment with ranitidine compared with fundoplication in gastro-oesophageal reflux disease. Scand J Gastroenterol 21: 779-788.

17. Klinkenberg-Knol EC (1992) The role of omeprazole in healing and prevention of reflux disease. Hepatogastroenterology 39 Suppl 1: 27-30.

18. Laursen LS, Havelund T, Bondesen S, et al. (1995) Omeprazole in the long-term treatment of gastro-oesophageal reflux disease. A double-blind randomized dose-finding study. Scand J Gastroenterol 30: 839-846.

19. Lundell LR (1994) The knife or the pill in the long-term treatment of gastroesophageal reflux disease? Yale J Biol Med 67: 233-246.

20. Lundell L, Backman L, Ekstrom P, et al. (1990) Omeprazole or high-dose ranitidine in the treatment of patients with reflux oesophagitis not responding to 'standard doses' of H2-receptor antagonists. Aliment Pharmacol Ther 4: 145-155.

21. Marks RD, Richter JE, Rizzo J, et al. (1994) Omeprazole versus H2-receptor antagonists in treating patients with peptic stricture and esophagitis. Gastroenterology 106: 907-915.

22. Mössner J, Hölscher AH, Herz R, Schneider A (1995) A double-blind study of pantoprazole and omeprazole in the treatment of reflux oesophagitis: a multicentre trial. Aliment Pharmacol Ther 9: 321-326.

23. Robertson CS, Evans DF, Ledingham SJ, Atkinson M (1993) Cisapride in the treatment of gastro-oesophageal reflux disease. Aliment Pharmacol Ther 7: 181-190.

24. Robinson M, Decktor DL, Maton PN, et al. (1993) Omeprazole is superior to ranitidine plus metoclopramide in the short-term treatment of erosive oesophagitis. Aliment Pharmacol Ther 7: 67-73.

25. Rush DR, Stelmach WJ, Young TL, et al. (1995) Clinical effectiveness and quality of life with ranitidine vs placebo in gastroesophageal reflux disease patients: a clinical experience network (CEN) study. J Fam Pract 41: 126-136.

26. Sandmark S, Carlsson R, Fausa O, Lundell L (1988) Omeprazole or ranitidine in the treatment of reflux esophagitis. Results of a double-blind, randomized, Scandinavian multicenter study. Scand J Gastroenterol 23: 625-632.

27. Smith PM, Kerr GD, Cockel R, et al. (1994) A comparison of omeprazole and ranitidine in the prevention of recurrence of benign esophageal stricture. Restore Investigator Group. Gastroenterology 107: 1312-1318.

28. Sontag SJ, Hirschowitz BI, Holt S, et al. (1992) Two doses of omeprazole versus placebo in symptomatic erosive esophagitis: the U.S. Multicenter Study. Gastroenterology 102: 109-118.

29. Toussaint J, Gossuin A, Deruyttere M, Huble F, Devis G (1991) Healing and prevention of relapse of reflux oesophagitis by cisapride. Gut 32: 1280-1285.

30. Tytgat GN, Anker Hansen OJ, Carling L, et al. (1992) Effect of cisapride on relapse of reflux oesophagitis, healed with an antisecretory drug. Scand J Gastroenterol 27: 175-183.

31. Vantrappen G, Rutgeerts L, Schurmans P, Coenegrachts JL (1988) Omeprazole (40 mg) is superior to ranitidine in short-term treatment of ulcerative reflux esophagitis. Dig Dis Sci 33: 523-529.
32. Vigneri S, Termini R, Leandro G, et al. (1995) A comparison of five maintenance therapies for reflux esophagitis. N Engl J Med 333: 1106-1110.
33. Zeitoun P, Rampal P, Barbier P, et al. (1989) [Omeprazole (20 mg daily) compared to ranitidine (150 mg twice daily) in the treatment of esophagitis caused by reflux. Results of a double-blind randomized multicenter trial in France and Belgium]. Gastroenterol Clin Biol 13: 457-462.
34. Watson DI, Pike GK, Baigrie RJ, et al. (1997) Prospective double-blind randomized trial of laparoscopic Nissen fundoplication with division and without division of short gastric vessels. Ann Surg 226: 642-652.
35. Luostarinen ME, Isolauri JO (1999) Randomized trial to study the effect of fundic mobilization on long-term results of Nissen fundoplication. Br J Surg 86: 614-618.
36. Laws HL, Clements RH, Swillie CM (1997) A randomized, prospective comparison of the Nissen fundoplication versus the Toupet fundoplication for gastroesophageal reflux disease. Ann Surg 225: 647-654.
37. Watson DI, Jamieson GG (1998) Antireflux surgery in the laparoscopic era. Br J Surg 85: 1173-1184.
38. Rydberg L, Ruth M, Abrahamsson H, Lundell L (1999) Tailoring antireflux surgery: A randomized clinical trial. World J Surg 23: 612-618.
39. Heikkinen TJ, Haukipuro K, Koivukangas P, et al. (1999) Comparison of costs between laparoscopic and open Nissen fundoplication: a prospective randomized study with a 3-month followup. J Am Coll Surg 188: 368-376.
40. Conference de consensus franco-belge (1999) Reflux gastro-oesophagien de l'adulte--diagnostic et traitement. Paris, France, 21-22 janvier 1999. Gastroenterol Clin Biol 23: S1-320.
41. Société Nationale Française de Gastro-Entérologie, Société Royale Belge de Gastro-Entérologie/Vlaamse Vereniging Voor Gastroenterologie, Société Française de Chirurgie Digestive, Société Française d'Endoscopie Digestive, Société Française de Pharmacologie (1999) Reflux gastro-oesophagien de l'adulte: "diagnostic et traitement". Conclusions et recommandations du jury: texte court. Gastroentérol Clin Biol 23: 66-71.
42. Fuchs KH, Feussner H, Bonavina L, Collard JM, Coosemans W (1997) Current status and trends in laparoscopic antireflux surgery: results of a consensus meeting. The European Study Group for Antireflux Surgery (ESGARS). Endoscopy 29: 298-308.
43. Moss SF, Arnold R, Tytgat GN, et al. (1998) Consensus Statement for Management of Gastroesophageal Reflux Disease: result of workshop meeting at Yale University School of Medicine, Department of Surgery, November 16 and 17, 1997. J Clin Gastroenterol 27: 6-12.

Diagnosis and treatment of common bile duct stones:

E.A.E.S. Consensus Development Conference (1997)[1,2] with updating comments (2000)

Conference organizers (1997):

A. PAUL, Surgical Clinic Merheim, 2nd Department of Surgery, University of Cologne (Germany);

B. MILLAT, Service de Chirurgie Viszerale A, Hôpital Saint Eloi, Montpellier (France);

U. HOLTHAUSEN, Surgical Clinic Merheim, 2nd Department of Surgery, University of Cologne (Germany);

S. SAUERLAND, Biochemical and Experimental Division, 2nd Department of Surgery, University of Cologne (Germany);

E. NEUGEBAUER, Biochemical and Experimental Division, 2nd Department of Surgery, University of Cologne (Germany);

Expert Panel (1997):

J. C. BERTHOU, Clinique chirurgicale mutualiste, Lorient (France);

H.-J. BRAMBS, Abteilung für Radiologie, University of Ulm (Germany);

J. E. DOMINGUEZ-MUÑOZ, Zentrum für Medizin, Otto-von-Guericke-Universität Magdeburg (Germany);

P. GOH, Department of Surgery, National University Hospital, Singapore (Singapore);

L. E. HAMMARSTRÖM, Department of Surgery, Malärsjukhuset, Eskilstuna (Sweden);

E. LEZOCHE, Cattedra di Chirugia Generale I, Universitá di Ancona (Italy);

J. PÉRISSAT, Service de Chirugie Digestive, Hopiteaux de Bordeaux (France);

1) Held at the 5th International Congress of the European Association for Endoscopic Surgery (E.A.E.S.), Istanbul, Turkey, 17-21 June, 1997
2) The original conference is published in Surg Endosc (1998) 12: 856-864.

P. Rossi, Istituto di Radiologia, Universitá degli Studi di Roma (Italy);

M. A. Röthlin, Klinik für Viszeralchirurgie, Universitätsspital Zürich (Switzerland);

R. C. G. Russell, Department of Surgery, Middlesex Hospital, London (United Kingdom);

P. Spinelli, Istituto Nazinale per lo Studio e la Cura dei Tumori, Milano (Italy);

Updating comments (2000):

A. Paul, Surgical Clinic Merheim, 2nd Department of Surgery, University of Cologne (Germany);

J. Treckmann, Surgical Clinic Merheim, 2nd Department of Surgery, University of Cologne (Germany)

Consensus statements (1997)

General Comment

Options for the management of common bile duct stones (CBDS) are increasing with the development of new technologies for diagnosis and treatment. While intraoperative cholangiography and open CBD exploration have comprised the applied technology for decades, the introduction of ERCP with endoscopic stone extraction in the 1970s and the more recent introduction of laparoscopic cholecystectomy led to a reappraisal of the situation. For each management policy, numerous publications - from case reports to prospective controlled clinical trials [1-42] - are available, but evidence-based conclusions can rarely be achieved yet.

In terms of predictors for CBDS, the crucial issue is perhaps not which indicators should best be applied to detect CBDS, but whether we should favor a high rate of negative examinations or a high rate of retained stones, with all their sequelae. The consequences of either strategy are currently not well understood and are often dependent on the local medical and nonmedical conditions. Nowadays, new imaging techniques in medicine, such as magnetic resonance cholangiopancreaticography (MRCP), have opened up new options for the diagnosis of CBDS. Furthermore, any debate about procedure and timing of diagnosis of CBDS leads to this question: Should they all be diagnosed?

Any discussion of an optimal therapy for common bile duct stones must take into account the rare but grave complications that each treatment option may entail. In general, the optimal diagnostic and therapeutic strategy seems to be dependent on local circumstances and the experience and expertise of the medical team, since there is still no evidence-based gold standard. In addition, ethical and socioeconomic considerations have an important impact on the controversy. For example, the costs of several techniques are prohibitive in some parts of the world.

Question 1. What are good indicators or predictive symptoms/signs for CBDS?

At the time of cholecystectomy for symptomatic cholelithiasis, 8-15% of patients under the age of 60 years and 15- 60% of patients over the age of 60 years have CBDS. This prevalence reflects the prior probability of any patient harboring CBDS before any discriminating test. The prevalence of CBDS has a decisive influence on the predictive value of any indicator. The prevalence of CBDS and the threshold for investigating CBDS vary among individual clinicians.

Among the many parameters investigated, no single indicator is completely accurate in predicting CBDS before cholecystectomy. The indicators can be grouped as follows: symptoms and signs, biochemical parameters, and imaging techniques. Although acute pancreatitis or cholecystitis are associated with a higher prevalence of CBDS, there is no good evidence that a history of pancreatitis is an indicator for CBDS.

Table 1 lists the predictive values for the main indicators of CBDS. These data were combined from several primary studies with a meta-analysis[43]. For each individual indicator, the lowest abnormal value is considered to be the threshold. Within a hypothetical population with symptomatic cholelithiasis, a 10% probability (prevalence) of harboring CBDS is assumed. As shown in the example in the table footnote, an individual patient's risk factors can be established by multiplying the relevant positive or negative likelihood ratios.

Table 1: Predictive values of preoperative indicators of CBDS (data from Abboud et al.[43], 1996, reprinted with permission)

Indicator	Sensitivity (95%-CI)	Specifity (95%-CI)	LR+	LR-
Cholangitis	0.11 (0.02-0.19)	0.99 (0.99-1.00)	18.3	0.93
Preop. jaundice	0.36 (0.26-0.45)	0.97 (0.95-0.99)	10.1	0.69
Cholecystitis	0.50 (0.11-0.89)	0.76 (0.45-1.00)	1.6	0.94
Biliruhine ↑	0.69 (0.48-0.90)	0.88 (0.84-0.92)	4.8	0.54
Alkaline Phosph ↑	0.57 (0.46-0.69)	0.86 (0.78-0.94)	2.6	0.65
Amylase ↑	0.11 (0.02-0.20)	0.95 (0.93-0.98)	1.5	0.99
CBDS on US	0.38 (0.27-0.49)	1.00 (0.99-1.00)	13.6	0.70
Dilated CBD on îUS	0.42 (0.28-0.56)	0.96 (0.94-0.98)	6.9	0.77

Data can be read as follows (line 1, cholangitis):
From 2% to 19% of patients with CBDS have cholangitis (defined as the triad pain-fever-jaundice). Nearly all patients who do not have CBDS also do not have cholangitis (column 2). A patient with CBDS is 18.3 times more likely to have cholangitis. If we assume prior odds to be 1 to 9 (i.e., 10% prevalence), we multiply 1/9 x 18.3 to get 2.03. So the posttest odds are about 2 to 1, which is a 66% probability. However, on the other hand, in a patient without CBDS (column 5), cholangitis is still not unlikely. We receive 1/9.67 posterior odds, or a 9.4% probability.
LR+ = positive Likelihood Ratio; LR- = negative Likelihood Ratio

A cystic duct found to have a diameter >4-5 mm at operation was associated with an increased probability of CBDS (sensitivity, 0.34; PPV, 0.52) in a population of 319 patients with a CBDS prevalence of 12% [12; 44].

In the clinical setting, several groups of patients can be identified, as follows: (a) **a high-risk group**, which fulfills a series of predictive factors resulting in a global probability of CBDS >90% based on the data in Table 1; (b) **a medium risk group**, or group of uncertainty, which fulfills one or several prognostic factors listed in Table 1 but for whom the resulting posttest probability (although higher than the pretest probability of 10%) does not reach 90%; (c) **a low-risk group**, which has no signs or symptoms. Although their probability of harboring CBDS is below average, in clinical practice unsuspected CBDS are found in £5% of patients with symptomatic gallbladder stones.

Question 2. Which diagnostic tools are useful in the detection of CBDS? In which order should they be applied?

Preoperative ultrasonography (US) misses two of three patients with common bile duct stones. However, it is a useful screening tool for the diagnosis of CBDS because of its noninvasiveness, easy availability, and low costs. Of all tools it should be applied as first. It has a reasonable predictive value if the CBD diameter is dilated as an indirect sign for CBDS. According to the literature, the sensitivity of preoperative US is 0.14-0.40, depending on the investigator's experience, the defined threshold value, and the general prevalence. The diagnosis of CBDS is more frequently achieved exclusively in patients with dilated CBD (diameter > 8-10 mm). Furthermore, liver or pancreas pathologies are also detectable by this means.

Preoperative Intravenous cholangiography (PIC) does not play a major role in the diagnosis of CBDS anymore. PIC has been reevaluated in patients without jaundice, using a new contrast reagent (meglumine iotroxate) with a reported risk of <1% adverse reactions. Infusion yields a satisfactory bile duct opacification in 90-95% of patients. The negative predictive value (NPV) of a normal PIC is 0.98-1. The positive predictive value (PPV) of PIC for CBDS diagnosis was 0.94 for stones demonstrated at PIC but only 0.31 for stones suspected at PIC. Previous studies showed that PIC missed CBDS in an average of 40% of cases (range, 22-90% sensitivity). Therefore, it is not recommended as a routine procedure. It may be an option based on the local circumstances of a center.

Endoscopic retrograde cholangiopancreatography (ERCP) is a valid diagnostic tool (high sensitivity, specificity, accuracy in experienced hands). It should only be applied with the intention to treat in patients with a high probability of CBDS who are eligible for ES. It has to be recognized that the procedure is invasive and inconvenient for the patient. It requires sedation and has defined morbidity (5-10%) and mortality (<1% for diagnostic purpose) rates. The success rate for ERCP is 95%. The sensitivity is 0.84-0.89. Specificity is 0.97-1. PPV is 1 and NPV is 0.88.

Endoscopic ultrasonography (EUS) is another exclusively diagnostic procedure with a high accuracy rate, but currently there is no indication for its routine use in diagnosing CBDS. The sensitivity of endoscopic ultrasound is 93%; specificity is 97%. PPV is 98% and NPV is 88%.

Intraoperative cholangiography (IOC) and **laparoscopic ultrasound** are reliable diagnostic tools (> 90% accuracy). Modern equipment and the use of fluoroscopy is required and may increase the accuracy in general practice. However, routine performance for the detection of symptomatic CBDS is questionable, although some of our panelists did recommend it. No final consensus was achieved regarding this point. The decision to perform routine or selective IOC during cholecystectomy depends both on the physician's personal beliefs regarding asymptomatic CBDS and his or her individual strategy for treatment. Reasons other than detection of CBDS for performing IOC, such as clarification of biliary anatomy, were considered outside the scope of the consensus. Invasive preoperative diagnostic tests should be avoided in patients scheduled for elective cholecystectomy.

Magnetic resonance cholangiopancreaticography (MRCP) seems to be an excellent diagnostic tool with high accuracy rates, so it might supersede other invasive diagnostic procedures such as ERCP. Disadvantages include inconvenience for the patient, low availability, and high costs. Furthermore, it is not applicable in every case (morbid obesity, pacemaker, etc.). In a first study from Italy, [45] MRCP showed 91.6% sensitivity, 100% specificity, and an overall diagnostic accuracy of 96.8%.

Computer tomography (CT) has been evaluated only in biased populations. It plays no role in routine management.

All patients with symptomatic gallbladder stones need to be assessed for CBDS, and the treatment of all diagnosed CBDS is mandatory (eight of 12 panelists were in favor of it). There are three options:

■ Routine IOC requires no preoperative screening for CBDS. The rate of useless examinations is in correspondence with the prevalence of CBDS in the population sheduled for cholecystectomy.

■ Selective contraindication for IOC is based on the negative predictive value of indicators for CBDS. It allows a 30-50% reduction in the number of IOC and yields a 2-3% rate of missed CBDS.

■ Selective indication for IOC is based on the positive predictive value of preoperative indicators for CBDS. It limits diagnosis and treatment exclusively to preoperatively symptomatic CBDS. Limitations are related to the information provided by the predictors and uncertainty regarding the natural history of asymptomatic CBDS.

Question 3. When should CBDS be diagnosed?

The timing of diagnostics should be dependent on the status of the patient and on the preferred treatment modality of the center,- pre- or intraoperatively. A routine policy of postoperative diagnoses of patients with a preoperative suspicion for CBDS is not advisable, since it entails the risk of a second operative intervention.

Question 4. Should CBDS be treated before, during or after cholecystectomy?

Depending on the clinical status of the patient, treatment can be performed before or during surgery. The policy of the specific center, as well as the experience and expertise of the medical team, may affect the choice of treatment modalities yet yield similar results. Postoperative treatment of CBDS is only necessary if intraoperative clearance of the common bile duct fails or if patients develop symptoms of retained stones.

Table 2: Results of 6 prospective randomised trials [2; 10; 23; 35; 37; 40] comparing preoperative ERC/ES versus open surgery alone for CBDS.

	Surgery	preop ERC/ES
Total number of patients included	302	283
Endoscopic failures		15 (5%)
Successful primary extraction	275 (91%)	233 (82%)
Complications (range)		
major	8% (4-15)	8% (4-10)
minor	15% (8-15)	10% (6-17)
total	23% (18-31)	19% (12-26)
Deaths	4 (1.3%)	8 (2.8%)
Residual stones (range)	4.9% (2-12)	3.4% (0-12)

Question 5. Which is the best treatment for CBDS and what is the appropriate surgical procedure for CBDS with gallbladder in situ?

There is no standard treatment today. In principle, three treatment regimens are available: endoscopic stone extraction during ERCP, laparoscopic and open bile duct exploration. There is no strong evidence from controlled trials that one procedure is superior to another in experienced hands. The majority of panel members saw no advantages of laparoscopic surgery over ERCP in terms of intraoperative safety, postoperative complications, mortality, pain, hospital stay, return to work, or cosmesis.

Laparoscopic bile duct exploration or a combination of endoscopic stone removal and laparoscopic cholecystectomy might be better compared to open surgery in terms of such aspects as less pain and faster recovery.

The laparoscopic transcystic approach and the laparoscopic choledochotomy are feasible. For ASA I/II patients, they might be preferable to preoperative ERCP and endoscopic sphincterotomy (ES) followed by laparoscopic cholecystectomy, since they shorten the duration of hospital stay.

Question 6. Treatment in special situations:

6a. Should asymptomatic CBDS be treated?

Because of the impredictibility of the occurence of symptoms or complications, diagnosed stones should be treated in all cases. It is additionally an ethical problem to knowingly leave stones behind. However, an expectant management for CBDS is acceptable in high-risk patients (ASA III/IV) and in patients unfit for surgery. These patients may benefit from endoscopic treatment alone.

6.b. Which is the appropriate treatment for large and/or impacted CBDS?

Large and/or impacted stones are a rare and ill-defined condition. Their treatment is usually difficult and depends on individual expertise. Options include:

- Endoscopic treatment (with the adjunct of lithotripsy)
- Primary surgery (laparoscopic or open approach with the adjunct of intraoperative lithotripsy and/or hepaticojejunostomy)
- Extracorporeal shockwave lithotripsy (ESWL) with or without ES.

6.c. How should CBDS in cholecystectomized patients be managed?

All patients with the described condition should be first treated by endoscopy, if feasible, including lithotripsy as required. There is as yet no evidence that endoscopic sphincterotomy or dilation of the sphincter performed in younger patients has a long-term negative outcome with higher rates of cholangitis, papillary stenosis, or other sequelae.

Question 7. Is cholecystectomy always compulsory in patients with CBDS?

Available data suggest that cholecystectomy should be recommended in patients with CBDS. In patient with major risk factors for surgery or in elderly patients, an individual management policy - e.g., leaving the gallbladder in-situ - can be justified. In Oriental cholangitis and in patients without gallbladder stones, cholecystectomy is usually not indicated after clearance of the common bile duct.

Question 8. What are the long-term results and sequelae of therapeutic interventions?

For both endoscopic sphincterotomy and open surgical common bile duct exploration, the long-term complication rates are reported to be in the same range (<10%), and the procedures have a high success rate in experienced hands. There are no data on the long-term complication rate of laparoscopic bile duct exploration.

Closing remarks:

■ The emerging success of MR cholangiopancreaticography, which has provided an excellent roadmap for the surgeon, should help to stem the debate over the diagnostic purpose of ERCP.

■ The general population of surgeons should be brought up to date about the technology of laparo-scopic bile duct exploration, furthermore, additional research is urgently needed.

■ There should be a follow-up of the results of this conference in the year 2000.

Updating comments (2000)

Introduction

In general, it remains to be uncertain what are the optimal diagnostic and therapeutic strategies for common bile duct stones. Personal expertise and experience of the surgical, medical, and radiology team and costs or socio-economy seem to be dominating factors still. It can be even speculated, that these factors while hopefully providing similar safety and efficacy are often overruling treatment endpoints such as "pain", "recovery", or "back to normal activity".

Although there is a clear trend in the last decade from large incisions towards "closed cavity" treatment options (laparoscopy and conventional interventional endoscopy), procedures such as laparoscopic common bile duct revisions are still not adapted by many surgeons. Possible reasons are that laparoscopic bile duct surgery involves demanding techniques, long learning curves even for otherwise well trained surgeons and inadequate instruments. Surgical training programs are often not well structured and new methods for training in endoscopic surgery still have to be developed and evaluated [46; 47]. Additionally specialization is already high and increasing, e.g. ERCP and endoscopic papillotomy (EPT) are rather performed by physicians, PTC(D) by interventional radiologists and not by surgeons. Therefore, an interdisciplinary team approach is usually necessary and overall success may depend on the strength of the team.

This update of the 1997 EAES Consensus Conference on Diagnosis and Treatment of CBDS is based on an extensive literature review using medline search of publications on CBDS published between 1997 and 1999. Only publications with grade III (controlled clinical trials) and grade II (sufficiently large prospective studies) were considered. However, this update is probably limited and biased by our methods of literature review and assessment and does not necessarily reflect the opinion of the initial panel.

Diagnosis of CBDS

The ongoing unsolved crucial issue in diagnosis and even treatment of CBDS is whether one should favor a high rate of negative examinations or a higher rate of retained stones. The benefit or harm of either strategy short and long term remains to be settled. Further studies [48; 49] underlined that cholangitis, dilated common bile duct with evidence of stones by ultrasound, elevated conjugated bilirubin, and less likely elevated asparate transaminase were predictive as individual factors and jointly excellent indicators (PPV 99%) for CBDS.

Conventional ultrasound continues to be a useful screening tool. Intravenous cholangiography is of very limited value and there are few studies indicating its routine use [50; 51]. Endoscopic retrograde cholangiopranicreatography (ERCP) provides an accuracy of at least > 90 % but seems to be indicated for diagnosis of CBDS when there is an intention to treat by EPT and stone extraction at the same session or when MRC or endoscopic ultrasound is not available. Alternatively CBDS are diagnosed intraoperatively by i.o.-cholangiography [52] or intraoperative ultrasound when single stage procedures are applied. Especially intraoperative ultrasound can have a very high accuracy (> 95 %) in specialized centers [52; 53].

Dependent on patient selection endoscopic ultrasound (EU) and magnetic resonance cholangipancreatiticography (MRCP) have sensitivity (> 95%) and specificity (> 90%) [54-58]. Both diagnostic tests require expensive technology, are operator dependent, and more or less inconvenient to the patient. However, especially technology of MRCP is rapidly evolving and is increasingly gaining acceptance. MRC(P) whenever available should be the standard diagnostic test in patients with medium or high risk for CBDS when EPT and stone extraction is not the possible or preferred method of treatment.

Treatment of CBDS

According to published (external) evidence there is no option which can be identified as the "standard treatment". Endoscopic stone extraction during ERCP, laparoscopic transcystic or laparoscopic common bile duct revision, and open duct exploration are applied. All three treatment options can be very effective and safe in experienced hands, however all three treatment principals have their specific disadvantages [59]. Depending on the study design some further arguments for laparoscopic bile duct revision [60] and for open common bile duct revision [61] have been published as a result of controlled trials.

Common bile duct stones following cholecystectomy should be primarily treated by endoscopy. In the absence of cholangitis indication for "routine" cholecystectomy after endoscopic duct clearance can be individualized in high risk patients.

In order to potentially reduce long term complications of endoscopic sphincterotomy endoscopic dilatation for stone clearance showed similar clearance rates, less bleeding, and preservation of sphincter function in controlled trials [3; 62; 63].

General comment

Due to inconclusiveness of published data and a high interpatient variability no clear cut recommendations for diagnosis and treatment of common bile duct stones can be given. We believe that less invasive and potentially less harmful procedures (e.g. MRCP versus ERCP for diagnosis, balloon dilatation versus endoscopic sphincterotomy for small stones) and procedures increasing the comfort of the patient (e.g. laparoscopic versus open common bile duct revision) should be more frequently applied and appropriately investigated. Training and continuous education should be intensified in academic institutions. New and more effective methods of training should be developed in these institutions.

References

(Ref. 1 – 45 relate to high-quality studies, which the original recommendations were based on. Ref. 46 – 63 are mainly high-quality studies but also commentaries published since then.)

1. Alinder G, Nilsson U, Lunderquist A, Herlin P, Holmin T (1986) Pre-operative infusion cholangiography compared to routine operative cholangiography at elective cholecystectomy. Br J Surg 73: 383-387.
2. Lenriot JP, Le Neel JC, Hay JM, et al. (1993) Cholangio-pancréatographie rétrograde et sphinctérotomie endoscopique pour lithiase biliaire. Évaluation prospective en milieu chirurgical. Gastroentérol Clin Biol 17: 244-250.
3. Bergman JJGHM, Rauws EAJ, Fockens P, et al. (1997) Randomised trial of endoscopic balloon dilation versus endoscopic sphincterotomy for removal of bileduct stones. Lancet 349: 1124-1129.
4. Canto MI, Chak A, Stellato T, Sivak MV, Jr. (1998) Endoscopic ultrasonography versus cholangiography for the diagnosis of choledocholithiasis. Gastrointest Endosc 47: 439-448.
5. Chopra KB, Peters RA, PA OT, et al. (1996) Randomised study of endoscopic biliary endoprosthesis versus duct clearance for bileduct stones in high-risk patients. Lancet 348: 791-793.
6. Cuschieri A, Croce E, Faggioni A, et al. (1996) EAES ductal stone study. Preliminary findings of multi-center prospective randomized trial comparing two-stage vs single-stage management. Surg Endosc 10: 1130-1135.

7. Daly J, Fitzgerald T, Simpson CJ (1987) Pre-operative intravenous cholangiography as an alternative to routine operative cholangiography in elective cholecystectomy. Clin Radiol 38: 161-163.
8. Duron JJ, Roux JM, Imbaud P, et al. (1987) Biliary lithiasis in the over seventy-five age group: a new therapeutic strategy. Br J Surg 74: 848-849.
9. Fölsch UR, Nitsche R, Lüdtke R, Hilgers RA, Creutzfeldt W (1997) Early ERCP and papillotomy compared with conservative treatment for acute biliary pancreatitis. The German Study Group on Acute Biliary Pancreatitis. N Engl J Med 336: 237-242.
10. Hammarström LE, Holmin T, Stridbeck H, Ihse I (1995) Long-term follow-up of a prospective randomized study of endoscopic versus surgical treatment of bile duct calculi in patients with gallbladder in situ. Br J Surg 82: 1516-1521.
11. Hauer-Jensen M, Kåresen R, Nygaard K, et al. (1986) Consequences of routine peroperative cholangiography during cholecystectomy for gallstone disease: a prospective, randomized study. World J Surg 10: 996-1002.
12. Hauer-Jensen M, Kåresen R, Nygaard K, et al. (1993) Prospective randomized study of routine intraoperative cholangiography during open cholecystectomy: long-term follow-up and multivariate analysis of predictors of choledocholithiasis. Surgery 113: 318-323.
13. Lacaine F, Corlette MB, Bismuth H (1980) Preoperative evaluation of the risk of common bile duct stones. Arch Surg 115: 1114-1116.
14. Lai ECS, Mok FPT, Tan ESY, et al. (1992) Endoscopic biliary drainage for severe acute cholangitis. N Engl J Med 326: 1582-1586.
15. Lai EC, Mok FP, Tan ES, et al. (1992) Endoscopic biliary drainage for severe acute cholangitis. N Engl J Med 326: 1582-1586.
16. Lewis RT, Allan CM, Goodall RG, et al. (1984) A single preoperative dose of cefazolin prevents postoperative sepsis in high-risk biliary surgery. Can J Surg 27: 44-47.
17. Liberman MA, Phillips EH, Carroll BJ, et al. (1996) Cost-effective management of complicated choledocholithiasis: laparoscopic transcystic duct exploration or endoscopic sphincterotomy. J Am Coll Surg 182: 488-494.
18. Lindsell DR (1990) Ultrasound imaging of pancreas and biliary tract. Lancet 335: 390-393.
19. Lygidakis NJ (1982) A prospective randomized study of recurrent choledocholithiasis. Surg Gynecol Obstet 155: 679-684.
20. Minami A, Nakatsu T, Uchida N, et al. (1995) Papillary dilation vs sphincterotomy in endoscopic removal of bile duct stones. A randomized trial with manometric function. Dig Dis Sci 40: 2550-2554.
21. Murison MS, Gartell PC, McGinn FP (1993) Does selective peroperative cholangiography result in missed common bile duct stones? J R Coll Surg Edinb 38: 220-224.
22. Neoptolemos JP, Carr-Locke DL, London NJ, et al. (1988) Controlled trial of urgent endoscopic retrograde cholangiopancreatography and endoscopic sphincterotomy versus conservative treatment for acute pancreatitis due to gallstones. Lancet 2: 979-983.
23. Neoptolemos JP, Carr-Locke DL, Fossard DP (1987) Prospective randomised study of preoperative endoscopic sphincterotomy versus surgery alone for common bile duct stones. Br Med J 294: 470-474.
24. Neoptolemos JP, Shaw DE, Carr-Locke DL (1989) A multivariate analysis of preoperative risk factors in patients with common bile duct stones. Implications for treatment. Ann Surg 209: 157-161.
25. Neuhaus H, Ungeheuer A, Feussner H, Classen M, Siewert JR (1992) Laparoskopische Cholezystektomie: ERCP als präoperative Standarddiagnostik? Dtsch Med Wochenschr 117: 1863-1867.
26. Panis Y, Fagniez PL, Brisset D, et al. (1993) Long term results of choledochoduodenostomy versus choledochojejunostomy for choledocholithiasis. The French Association for Surgical Research. Surg Gynecol Obstet 177: 33-37.
27. Ponchon T, Bory R, Chavaillon A, Fouillet P (1989) Biliary lithiasis: combined endoscopic and surgical treatment. Endoscopy 21: 15-18.
28. Röthlin MA, Schlumpf R, Largiadèr F (1994) Laparoscopic sonography. An alternative to routine intraoperative cholangiography? Arch Surg 129: 694-700.

29. Röthlin MA, Schöb O, Schlumpf R, Largiadèr F (1996) Laparoscopic ultrasonography during cholecystectomy. Br J Surg 83: 1512-1516.
30. Seifert E, Gail K, Weismüller J (1982) Langzeitresultate nach endoskopischer Sphinkterotomie. Dtsch Med Wochenschr 107: 610-614.
31. Sheen-Chen SM, Chou FF (1995) Intraoperative choledochoscopic electrohydraulic lithotripsy for difficulty retrieved impacted common bile duct stones. Arch Surg 130: 430-432.
32. Sigel B, Machi J, Beitler JC, et al. (1983) Comparative accuracy of operative ultrasonography and cholangiography in detecting common duct calculi. Surgery 94: 715-720.
33. Soper NJ, Dunnegan DL (1992) Routine versus selective intra-operative cholangiography during laparoscopic cholecystectomy. World J Surg 16: 1133-1140.
34. Soto JA, Barish MA, Yucel EK, et al. (1996) Magnetic resonance cholangiography: comparison with endoscopic retrograde cholangiopancreatography. Gastroenterology 110: 589-597.
35. Stain SC, Cohen H, Tsuishoysha M, Donovan AJ (1991) Choledocholithiasis. Endoscopic sphincterotomy or common bile duct exploration. Ann Surg 213: 627-633; discussion 633-624.
36. Stark ME, Loughry CW (1980) Routine operative cholangiography with cholecystectomy. Surg Gynecol Obstet 151: 657-658.
37. Stiegmann GV, Goff JS, Mansour A, et al. (1992) Precholecystectomy endoscopic cholangiography and stone removal is not superior to cholecystectomy, cholangiography, and common duct exploration. Am J Surg 163: 227-230.
38. Stoker ME (1995) Common bile duct exploration in the era of laparoscopic surgery. Arch Surg 130: 265-268; discussion 268-269.
39. Tanaka M, Sada M, Eguchi T, et al. (1996) Comparison of routine and selective endoscopic retrograde cholangiography before laparoscopic cholecystectomy. World J Surg 20: 267-270; discussion 271.
40. Targarona EM, Perez Ayuso RM, Bordas JM, et al. (1996) Randomised trial of endoscopic sphincterotomy with gallbladder left in situ versus open surgery for common bileduct calculi in high-risk patients. Lancet 347: 926-929.
41. Wermke W, Schulz HJ (1987) Sonographische Diagnostik von Gallenwegskonkrementen. Ultraschall Med 8: 116-120.
42. Kapoor R, Kaushik SP, Saraswat VA, et al. (1996) Prospective randomized trial comparing endoscopic sphincterotomy followed by surgery with surgery alone in good risk patients with choledocholithiasis. HPB Surg 9: 145-148.
43. Abboud PA, Malet PF, Berlin JA, et al. (1996) Predictors of common bile duct stones prior to cholecystectomy: a meta-analysis. Gastrointest Endosc 44: 450-455.
44. Hauer-Jensen M, Kåresen R, Nygaard K, et al. (1985) Predictive ability of choledocholithiasis indicators. A prospective evaluation. Ann Surg 202: 64-68.
45. Lomanto D, Pavone P, Laghi A, et al. (1997) Magnetic resonance-cholangiopancreatography in the diagnosis of biliopancreatic diseases. Am J Surg 174: 33-38.
46. Hamdorf JM, Hall JC (2000) Acquiring surgical skills. Br J Surg 87: 28-37.
47. Troidl H (1999) Wie bekomme ich einen guten Chirurgen? Wie werde ich ein guter Chirurg? Zentralbl Chir 124: 868-875.
48. Alponat A, Kum CK, Rajnakova A, Koh BC, Goh PM (1997) Predictive factors for synchronous common bile duct stones in patients with cholelithiasis. Surg Endosc 11: 928-932.
49. Trondsen E, Edwin B, Reiertsen O, et al. (1998) Prediction of common bile duct stones prior to cholecystectomy: a prospective validation of a discriminant analysis function. Arch Surg 133: 162-166.
50. Nies C, Bauknecht F, Groth C, et al. (1997) Intraoperative Cholangiographie als Routinemethode? Eine prospektive, kontrollierte, randomisierte Studie. Chirurg 68: 892-897.
51. Holzinger F, Baer HU, Wildi S, Vock P, Büchler MW (1999) Die Rolle der intravenösen Cholangiographie im Zeitalter der laparoskopischen Cholezystektomie: Eine Renaissance? Dtsch Med Wochenschr 124: 1373-1378.

52. Siperstein A, Pearl J, Macho J, et al. (1999) Comparison of laparoscopic ultrasonography and fluorocholangiography in 300 patients undergoing laparoscopic cholecystectomy. Surg Endosc 13: 113-117.
53. Birth M, Ehlers KU, Delinikolas K, Weiser HF (1998) Prospective randomized comparison of laparoscopic ultrasonography using a flexible-tip ultrasound probe and intraoperative dynamic cholangiography during laparoscopic cholecystectomy. Surg Endosc 12: 30-36.
54. Demartines N, Eisner L, Schnabel K, et al. (2000) Evaluation of magnetic resonance cholangiography in the management of bile duct stones. Arch Surg 135: 148-152.
55. Zidi SH, Prat F, Le Guen O, et al. (1999) Use of magnetic resonance cholangiography in the diagnosis of choledocholithiasis: prospective comparison with a reference imaging method. Gut 44: 118-122.
56. Hintze RE, Adler A, Veltzke W, et al. (1997) Clinical significance of magnetic resonance cholangiopancreatography (MRCP) compared to endoscopic retrograde cholangiopancreatography (ERCP). Endoscopy 29: 182-187.
57. de Ledinghen V, Lecesne R, Raymond JM, et al. (1999) Diagnosis of choledocholithiasis: EUS or magnetic resonance cholangiography? A prospective controlled study. Gastrointest Endosc 49: 26-31.
58. Montariol T, Msika S, Charlier A, et al. (1998) Diagnosis of asymptomatic common bile duct stones: preoperative endoscopic ultrasonography versus intraoperative cholangiography--a multicenter, prospective controlled study. Surgery 124: 6-13.
59. Cuschieri A, Lezoche E, Morino M, et al. (1999) E.A.E.S. multicenter prospective randomized trial comparing two-stage vs single-stage management of patients with gallstone disease and ductal calculi. Surg Endosc 13: 952-957.
60. Rhodes M, Sussman L, Cohen L, Lewis MP (1998) Randomised trial of laparoscopic exploration of common bile duct versus postoperative endoscopic retrograde cholangiography for common bile duct stones. Lancet 351: 159-161.
61. Suc B, Escat J, Cherqui D, et al. (1998) Surgery vs endoscopy as primary treatment in symptomatic patients with suspected common bile duct stones: a multicenter randomized trial. Arch Surg 133: 702-708.
62. Ido K, Tamada K, Kimura K, et al. (1997) The role of endoscopic balloon sphincteroplasty in patients with gallbladder and bile duct stones. J Laparoendosc Adv Surg Tech A 7: 151-156.
63. Ochi Y, Mukawa K, Kiyosawa K, Akamatsu T (1999) Comparing the treatment outcomes of endoscopic papillary dilation and endoscopic sphincterotomy for removal of bile duct stones. J Gastroenterol Hepatol 14: 90-96.

Diagnosis and treatment of diverticular disease:

E.A.E.S. Consensus Development Conference (1997)[1,2] with updating comments (2000)

Conference organizers (1998):

L. KÖHLER, Surgical Clinic Merheim, 2nd Department of Surgery, University of Cologne (Germany);
S. SAUERLAND, Biochemical and Experimental Division, 2nd Department of Surgery, University of Cologne (Germany);
E. NEUGEBAUER, Biochemical and Experimental Division, 2nd Department of Surgery, University of Cologne (Germany);

Expert Panel (1998):

R. CAPRILLI, Department of Gastroenterology, Università degli studi di Roma "La sapienza", Roma (Italy);
A. FINGERHUT, Centre Hospitalier Intercommunal, Poissy (France);
N. Y. HABOUBI, Department of Histopathology, Withington Hospital, Manchester (U.K.);
L. HULTÉN, Department of Surgery II, Sahlgrenska Sjukhuset, Göteborg (Sweden);
C. G. S. HÜSCHER, Divisione di Diagnostica e Chirurgie Endoscopica, Istituto Nazionale per lo Studio e la Cura dei Tumori, Milano (Italy);
A. JANSEN, Department of Surgery, Kennemer Gasthuis, Haarlem (Netherlands);
H.-U. KAUCZOR, Klinik und Poliklinik für Radiologie, J.-Gutenberg-Universität Mainz, Mainz (Germany);
M. R. KEIGHLEY, Department of Surgery, Queen Elizabeth Hospital, Birmingham (U.K.);
F. KÖCKERLING, Surgical Clinic "Siloah", Hannover (Germany);

1) Held at the 6nd International Congress of the European Association for Endoscopic Surgery (E.A.E.S.), Rome, Italy, May 31 – June 6, 1998
2) The original conference is published in Surg Endosc (1999) 13: 430-436.

W. KRUIS, Department of Gastroenterology, Evangelisches Krankenhaus Kalk, Köln (Germany);

A. LACY, Department of Surgery, Hospital Clínic, Barcelona (Spain);

K. LAUTERBACH, Institut für Gesundheitsökonomie und klinische Epidemiologie, Universität zu Köln, Köln (Germany);

J. LEROY, Department of Digestive Surgery, Digestive Cancer Research Institute (IRCAD) and European Institute of Telesurgery (EITS), Strasbourg (France);

J. M. MÜLLER, Department of Surgery, Charité, Humboldt-Universität, Berlin (Germany);

H. E. MYRVOLD, Department of Surgery, Trondheim University Hospital, Trondheim (Norway);

P. SPINELLI, Divisione di Diagnostica e Chirurgie Endoscopica, Istituto Nazionale per lo Studio e la Cura dei Tumori, Milano (Italy)

Updating comments (2000):

L. KÖHLER, Department of Surgery, Kreiskrankenhaus Grevenbroich - St.Elisabeth, Grevenbroich (Germany);

Consensus statements (1997)

1. Definition

In the literature, there is as yet no uniform definition of diverticular disease. Consensus in the following terminology was achieved:

Colonic diverticular disease is a condition seen mostly in the sigmoid region. It is characterized structurally by mucosal herniation through the colonic wall, generally accompanied by muscular thickening, elastosis of the taenia coli and mucosal folding.

This condition may be asymptomatic (**diverticulosis**) or associated with "symptoms", termed **diverticular disease**, which may be complicated or uncomplicated. The term **diverticulitis** is used to indicate superadded inflammation involving the bowel wall. Other pathologic complications include perforation, fistula, obstruction and bleeding.

2. Natural History

Colonic diverticulosis is an increasingly common condition. About a third of the population is affected by the sixth decade and a half by the ninth decade. The incidence of diverticular disease varies around 10 patients/100.000/year. About 200.000 admissions to hospital in the USA annually are due to diverticular disease. The sex predilection has changed during the century from a male to a female predominance. It is well documented that the disease is more common in Western Societies rather than in the Developing World, which has been explained by the etiology of the disease. In Eastern Asia right-side colonic diverticula or bilateral disease has been found to be more common.

The **natural history** is not very well investigated within prospective studies. No good indicators are available to distinguish the patients who will become symptomatic from those who will not.

3. Etiology

The etiology of diverticular disease is generally accepted as being associated with a lifelong **deficiency on dietary fiber**. It is believed that such a diet results in a small stool, the propulsion of which requires a high intracolonic pressure (equivalent to ≥ 150 mmHg). At the vulnerable regions where blood vessels enter the colonic wall, herniation is caused. Muscular thickening and elastosis of the taenia coli have also been documented.

A high roughage diet, such as tthat consumed by vegetarians, protects against diverticular disease. This type of diet offers an opportunity for primary disease prevention. In Western Countries, however, the decline of dietary fiber intake, mainly from cereal grains, resulted in a high disease prevalence, in sharp contrast with data from developing countries.

Aging is associated with a decreased tensile strength of both collagen and muscle fibers of the colon. In diverticulosis, similar changes occur, but exceed the effect ascribed to aging alone. Nevertheless, with increasing age the prevalence of diverticular disease rises steadily. Moderate and vigorous **physical activity** stimulates bowel activity and therefore may have a protective effect, at least in men. As **obesity** correlates with low physical activity levels and low fiber intake, it is associated with diverticular disease, but plays no causal role.

Some **hereditary diseases**, such as polycystic kidney disease, Marfan's and Ehlers-Danlos-syndrome, are associated with an increased disease incidence, since these diseases impair the strength of the submucosa. **Smoking** may modestly increase the risk of deloping diverticular disease. **Alcohol** and **caffeine** consumption do not play major roles in the etiology. **Immunosuppressed patients** (mainly transplant recipients) have an increased susceptibility to complicated diverticular disease.

Acute attacks of diverticulitis may be associated with hard feces becoming trapped in a diverticulum, causing mucosal ulceration and bacterial migration into the surrounding pericolic fat.

4. Classification

Diverticular disease can be classified with regard to the following aspects of the disease: localization, distribution, clinical symtoms and presentation, and pathology. Two classifications are of importance: the clinical classification and the Hinchey classification.

Clinical classification:

Subjective disease is difficult to grade, we consider crampy pain, fever, and subjective patients evaluations to be symptomatic. Disease is classified as follows:
- symptomatic uncomplicated disease
- recurrent symptomatic disease
- complicated disease (hemorrhage, abscess, phlegmon, perforation, purulent and fecal peritonitis, stricture, fistula, small bowel obstruction due to postinflammatory adhesions).

The modified Hinchey-classification should be used to describe the clinical stages of perforated diverticular disease:
- Stage I: Pericolic abscess
- Stage IIa: Distant abscess amenable to percutaneous drainage
- Stage IIb: Complex abscess associated with/without fistula

- Stage III: Generalized purulent peritonitis
- Stage IV: Fecal peritonitis

However, neither classification is validated according to established criteria.

5. Diagnosis

The choice in diagnostic procedures depends on clinical presentation. Differential diagnosis in coexisting intestinal disease has to be considered. First step of diagnosis is a history with respect of type, severity, and course of the symptoms. The second step may require barium enema, colonoscopy, laboratory tests, CT, sonography, or radiography. The order of the procedures depends on the clinical decision and the availability of the methods.

In **uncomplicated cases**, a colonoscopy with biopsy and/or a barium enema is necessary to rule out adenoma, carcinoma, colitis, and Crohn's disease. There is no consensus on which method should be used first, or whether biopsy is mandatory or recommended.

Patients with **recurrent symptomatic disease** who are eligible for surgery, especially if an endoscopic procedure is planned, should undergo CT and/or barium enema to provide information on location of the disease process, extraluminal changes, and co-existing abdominal abnormalities.

In **complicated diverticular disease** (except bleeding) cross-sectional imaging such as CT should be used in addition to plain abdominal radiography. CT has been reported to have an >90% sensitivity and specificity. Ultrasonography may serve as another good diagnostic tool, but depends on the experience of the examiner. If CT is unavailable or does not yield a conclusive diagnosis, a low-pressure, water-soluble contrast enema can be considered. Flexible endoscopy is not recommended in suspected perforation or abscess formation, since it may perforate the colonic wall. The value of magnetic resonance imaging (MRI) has yet not be studied in acute diverticular disease and should therefore be considered as experimental.

Cases of **acute obstructive diverticular disease** should be evaluated by water-soluble contrast enema to confirm the obstruction. If the patient has a chronic obstructive situation colonoscopy with biopsy should be performed.

In cases presenting with **massive bleeding**, a number of different approaches have been used successfully, including selective arteriography, endoscopy, and radionuclided scans. However, there is no consensus on which of the diagnostic tools is preferable as a first choice.

6. Criteria for making the treatment decision

There is consensus that **disease dependent criteria** for treatment decision include number of previous attacks, fever, anemia, leukocytosis, intraluminal narrowing, obstruction, fistulas, abscess formation, free air, intraabdominal fluid, and thickening of the wall verified by CT scan.

Patient dependent criteria include age and concomitant disease, functional and emotional status, degree of disability, cognitive function, and subjective well-being of the patient. However, these criteria have not been adequately considered in previous trials. The number of diverticula, their distribution, and manometry data should have no influence on decision making.

7. Indication for conservative treatment

There is a consensus that conservative treatment is indicated in cases with a first attack of uncomplicated diverticular disease. The rationale is that 50-70% of patients treated for a first episode of acute diverticulitis will recover and will have no further problems. Only about 20% of patients with a first attack develop any complications. Those with recurrent attacks are at 60% risk to develop complications. The members agreed that a detailed description of conservative treatment was outside the scope of the consensus conference. Appropriate conservative therapy of an attack of diverticular disease in mild cases consists of oral hydration, oral antibiotics (i.e., ciprofloxacin and metronidazol) and antispasmodics. In moderate or severe cases, oral feeding should be stopped to allow bowel rest. Hydration and anibiotics should be given intravenously. Analgesics can be given as required, including narcotics, but morphine should be avoided because of its potential to cause colonic spasm and hypersegmentation.

Patients with diverticular disease who are not suffering from an acute attack should be instructed to maintain a diet high in fiber. In patients who continue to experience some discomfort (such as mild cramps, meteorism, or stool irregularities) may benefit from the addition of bulking agents (i.e., plantago) or antispasmodics.

8. Indication for operative treatment

There is a consensus that prophylactic sigmoid colectomy is not justified in asymptomatic patients who have no history of inflammatory attacks. There is also agreement that prophylactic sigmoid colectomy should not be performed for symptomatic diverticular disease in the belief that complications would be prevented thereby. Patients should be considered for elective surgery, if they have had at least two attacks of symptomatic diverticular disease. No data on the significance of the timing and severity of an attack exist. The decision should be made by the treating doctor. At the same time, the benefits of resection for recurrent symptoms must be weighed against the risks of surgery in old, fragile patients and those with concurrent disease. This situation must be fully explained to patients (consensus). Surgery may be also indicated after the first attack in patients who require chronic immuno-suppression. Chronic complications like colovesicular or colovaginal fistulas, stenoses and bleeding are further indications for operation. If a concomitant carcinoma cannot excluded, surgery is also recommended.

9. Type of operation

For **symptomatic, uncomplicated disease,** there is a consensus that the diseased segment – usually the sigmoid colon - should be resected. The sigmoid myotomy is nowadays an outmoded procedure. It is not necessary to remove all diverticula. The distal resection line is just below the level of the rectosigmoid junction, and anastomosis is performed with the proximal rectum to prevent recurrent disease. The extent to be resected in oral direction is controversial. Many surgeons claim that the colon should be divided when the bowel is soft, even in the presence of diverticulae, while others suggest complete proximal resection of macroscopically involved bowel to achieve normal wall thickness without diverticula at the line of resection. There are insufficient data to resolve this issue. The left ureter should always be identified before resection is performed. During resection, the presacral nerves should be identified and preserved from damage.

Hinchey I (abscess confined to mesentery) should first be treated by percutaneous drainage where possible and then by sigmoid colectomy and primary anastomosis in fit patients (consensus).

Hinchey II (pelvic abscess, whatever the localisation) should also be treated by percutaneous drainage, and followed later by by sigmoid resection in most cases, but risk in patients with comorbidity must be considered in the final decision (consensus).

Hinchey III (purulent peritonitis) is a problematic situation: There are no valid data regarding best treatment. Options include Hartmann resection, or resection with primary anastomosis with or without a covering stoma. There is a need for randomized trials here (consensus).

Hinchey IV (fecal peritonitis) should be treated by the Hartmann procedure after rigorous preoperative resuscitation measures. Drainage alone by open operation is not viable for Hinchey III and IV (consensus).

Patients should be informed that the chance of restoring intestinal continuity is only 60% at best after a Hartmann procedure. Open surgery to rejoin the Hartmann operation is a major undertaking, and it is with a high potential for complications. (consensus).

If the **continuous and severe bleeding** is caused by diverticular disease, the involved segment should be resected. On-table lavage and endoscopy should be considered to localize the bleeding. However, exact localisation is often impossible. In these cases subtotal colectomy with ileorectal anastomosis is indicated. Selective intrarterial infusion of vasopressin and endoscoic injections hemostasis have been shown to be effective, but elective surgery should be considered to prevent recuirrence in the long term.

10. Place of laparoscopic procedures

There is a consensus that laparoscopic sigmoid resection may be an acceptable alternative to conventional sigmoid resection in patients with recurrent symptomatic disease or stenosis (for procedures, see Appendix). In Hinchey I and II patients, the laparoscopic approach is not the first choice, but it may be justified if no gross abnormalities are found during diagnostic laparoscopy. In some patients, peritoneal lavage or drainage of a localised abscess can be undertaken by laparoscopy.

There is no place today for laparoscopic resections in Hinchey III (diverticulitis with purulent peritonitis) and Hinchey IV (diverticulitis with fecal peritonitis). Laparoscopic hookup after a Hartmann resection may reduce morbidity, but there may be a high conversion rate.

All surgeons engaged in laparoscopic-assisted sigmoid colectomy must have a low threshold for converting to an open operation if difficulties are encountered or if the anatomy of the abdomen and pelvis cannot be clearly defined. The procedures should be restricted to surgeons experienced in laparoscopic techniques.

11. Laparoscopic technique

The aim of laparoscopic surgery is to minimize the surgical trauma. The same principles as in conventional surgery have to be applied in the laparoscopic technique.

12. Avoiding recurrent disease

In uncomplicated non-operated cases, recurrent attacks can be prevented by bulking agents, such as plantago. During the operation, the proper height of the proximal resection of the diseased bowel is still a controversial topic. The distal resection should be performed to the level of the rectum, where the taenia disappears. A specimen of ≥ 20 cm should be resected.

13. Long-term results and sequelae of therapeutic interventions

In **uncomplicated disease**, the data indicate that high-fiber diet provides symptomatic relief and protects from complications (<1% per patient year follow-up).

In **complicated disease**, after successful conservative treatment, the risk of further episodes of complications is £2% per patient year. Resection was required in £3% of patients in collected series.

Only few studies have focused on the outcome for the patients. Quality-of-life measurements are missing. Functional data concerning stool frequency, bowel habits, and continence after the operation are scarce. The persistence of intermittent pain in the lower abdomen after sigmoid resection is surprisingly high (1-27%).

14. Economics

Extensive literature reviews have turned up very little in the way of economic data on the treatment of diverticular disease, especially data that would allow a comparison of treatment options. We recommend that choice of treatment not be based on economic data currently, because costs may vary from one locale ot another. Further studies in this area are indicated.

Appendix: Laparoscopic sigmoidectomy

The patient is positioned in a modified Trendelenburg position. The pneumoperitoneum should not exceed a pressure of 12 mm Hg. Usually, four trocars are used, but more trocars can be used in cases of difficulties. The optic trocar is inserted above the umbilicus in the midline. Another 5- or 10-mm trocar is positioned in the left lower quadrant and two further trocars (10- and 12-mm) are placed in the lower right quadrant.

The dissection begins in the basis of the mesosigmoid, where the vessels are located and divided after identification of the left ureter. Some surgeons prefer the primary mobilization of the sigmoid colon after identification of the left ereter; others prefer to ligate the superior rectal artey or dissect even closer to the bowel. The mesenteric attachments are freed widely. The parietal peritoneum is divided up to the splenic flexure. Mobilizing the splenic flexure may be useful in creating a tension-free suture. After presacral nerves are identified, the rectosigmoid junction is divided by stapler. A mini-laparotomy is performed in the left lower quadrant, or a Pfannenstiel incision is done. The bowel is extracted through the mini-laparotomy and proximal resection is completed. Some surgeons use a bag to remove the specimen. The anvil of the stapling device is placed after performing a purse-string suture. After reestablishing the pneumoperitoneum, the stapler is introduced per-anally, and the anastomosis is completed. The completeness of the resection ring has to be examined. Integrity of the anastomosis is checked either by endoscope, or by methylene blue-colored water. Drainage of the pelvis is facultative.

Updating comments (2000)

Introduction

The consensus development conference on diverticular disease is the youngest of all CDCs organized by the E.A.E.S. Only nine month have passed since its publication. Many papers have been published on the pros and cons of laparoscopic surgery for the treatment of diverticular disease since 1998, but randomized clinical trials are still missing. New papers concerning the natural history of the disease are also scarce and the pathophysiology of diverticular disease is still not well understood, even though the disease is common in Western countries.

In the following paragraphs, the author will give an overview over the new data on the surgical therapy of diverticular disease. Laparoscopic sigmoid resection will be assessed by using technology assessment techniques as described by Jennett [1], and Frazier and Mosteller [2]. These criteria include (in a stepwise order): feasibility, efficacy, effectiveness, and cost efficiency.

Feasibility

The feasibility of laparoscopic sigmoid resection has been demonstrated in several studies [3-32], but technical performance is demanding, particular in cases with a long history of recurrent inflammatory disease. Compared to conventional sigmoid resection operative time may be prolonged, but by getting more and more experience it will be shorter [14]. Conversion rate is in between 5-20%, but depends on the experience of the surgeon and patient selection.

Bennett et al. [4] demonstrated that laparoscopy-assisted colectomy cases performed by high-volume surgeons are more likely to have better intraoperative and postoperative outcomes than cases performed by low-volume surgeons. Their data suggest that for this laparoscopic procedure there is a learning curve, and that about 40 cases are required to achieve good outcomes for colorectal procedures compared with only 20 for laparoscopic cholecystectomy.

In a very recent paper Schwandner et al. [33] demonstrated that risk factors contributing to the possibility of conversion include male gender, age between 55 and 64 years, extreme body status, and diverticular disease. However, if conversion is necessary, laparoscopic colorectal surgery can be safely applied to the patients with no additional morbidity. Their data are in contrast to the early data of Slim et al. [34], who demonstrated an increased morbidity after conversion. They concluded that careful preoperative patient selection for laparoscopic procedures and a rapid decision to convert in case of difficulty are important.

The disease-specific short-term goal of laparoscopic assisted sigmoid resection for the treatment of diverticular disease is achieved. The inflamed bowel is resected and the length of the resected bowel does not differ between both techniques [15].

However, all statements in regard of feasibility of laparoscopic sigmoid resection are only based on controlled studies without randomisation and descriptive studies such as comparative studies. Thus, the category of evidence as defined by AHCPR is IIa-III.

Efficacy

Compared to conventional techniques the mortality is equally low. Low grade morbidity is slightly reduced, and high grade morbidity is equally low. Several studies [3-32] have demonstrated a quicker postoperative recovery for laparoscopically treated patients, and the time of hospital stay is reduced. Patients experience less pain and better cosmesis. In the long term the incidence of incisional hernias may be reduced. Until now, however, it is not known if disease- specific long- term goals are achieved owing to the short follow-up time. The grade of evidence of all these statements is IIa according to the AHCPR.

A recently published German multicenter trial [35] confirms these statements and demonstrated that laparoscopic colorectal interventions in sigmoid diverticulitis are mainly carried out as elective procedures for peridiverticulitis, stenosis, or recurrent attacks of inflammation. The conversion, complication, and mortality rates associated with these interventions are acceptable. Laparoscopic procedures in perforated diverticular disease and in the presence of fistula and bleeding are at higher risk, and should be carried out only by highly experienced laparoscopic surgeons.

Effectiveness

Until now, wide applicability of the laparoscopic technique is not given, even though the laparoscopic resection rate may be high in specialised centers. However, we are very early in the evolution of laparoscopic colorectal surgery and the assessment may be invalid. The difference between the special expert and the average surgeon may continue long after endoscopic surgery has passed the stage of innovation.

Cost efficiency

The costs of health care delivery have become more and more important. Cost-benefit and cost-effectiveness analyses after laparoscopic and conventional sigmoid resection for diverticular disease are still missing. However, cost calculations demonstrate that laparoscopic sigmoid resection is not much more expensive compared than the conventional technique [6; 15; 18; 36].

References

1. Jennett B, Technology assessment - a question of information. In: High technology medicine. Benefits and burdens. Oxford University Press, Oxford/UK, 1986, pp. 227-231.
2. Frazier HS, Mosteller F, Medicine worth paying for: Assessing medical innovations., Harvard University Press, Cambridge/MA, 1995
3. Begos DG, Arsenault J, Ballantyne GH (1996) Laparoscopic colon and rectal surgery at a VA hospital. Analysis of the first 50 cases. Surg Endosc 10: 1050-1056.
4. Bennett CL, Stryker SJ, Ferreira MR, Adams J, Beart RW, Jr. (1997) The learning curve for laparoscopic colorectal surgery. Preliminary results from a prospective analysis of 1194 laparoscopic-assisted colectomies. Arch Surg 132: 41-45.

5. Bergamaschi R, Arnaud JP (1997) Immediately recognizable benefits and drawbacks after laparoscopic colon resection for benign disease. Surg Endosc 11: 802-804.
6. Bruce CJ, Coller JA, Murray JJ, et al. (1996) Laparoscopic resection for diverticular disease. Dis Colon Rectum 39: S1-6.
7. Eijsbouts QA, Cuesta MA, de Brauw LM, Sietses C (1997) Elective laparoscopic-assisted sigmoid resection for diverticular disease. Surg Endosc 11: 750-753.
8. Falk PM, Beart RW, Jr., Wexner SD, et al. (1993) Laparoscopic colectomy: a critical appraisal. Dis Colon Rectum 36: 28-34.
9. Fowler DL, White SA (1991) Laparoscopy-assisted sigmoid resection. Surg Laparosc Endosc 1: 183-188.
10. Franklin ME, Jr., Ramos R, Rosenthal D, Schuessler W (1993) Laparoscopic colonic procedures. World J Surg 17: 51-56.
11. Gellman L, Salky B, Edye M (1996) Laparoscopic assisted colectomy. Surg Endosc 10: 1041-1044.
12. Hotokezaka M, Dix J, Mentis EP, Minasi JS, Schirmer BD (1996) Gastrointestinal recovery following laparoscopic vs open colon surgery. Surg Endosc 10: 485-489.
13. Jacobs M, Verdeja JC, Goldstein HS (1991) Minimally invasive colon resection (laparoscopic colectomy). Surg Laparosc Endosc 1: 144-150.
14. Köhler L, Holthausen U, Troidl H (1997) Laparoskopische colorektale Chirurgie - Versuch der Bewertung einer neuen Technologie. Chirurg 68: 794-800.
15. Köhler L, Rixen D, Troidl H (1998) Laparoscopic colorectal resection for diverticulitis. Int J Colorectal Dis 13: 43-47.
16. Larach SW, Patankar SK, Ferrara A, et al. (1997) Complications of laparoscopic colorectal surgery. Analysis and comparison of early vs. latter experience. Dis Colon Rectum 40: 592-596.
17. Lacy AM, Garcia-Valdecasas JC, Pique JM, et al. (1995) Short-term outcome analysis of a randomized study comparing laparoscopic vs open colectomy for colon cancer. Surg Endosc 9: 1101-1105.
18. Liberman MA, Phillips EH, Carroll BJ, Fallas M, Rosenthal R (1996) Laparoscopic colectomy vs traditional colectomy for diverticulitis. Outcome and costs. Surg Endosc 10: 15-18.
19. Lumley JW, Fielding GA, Rhodes M, et al. (1996) Laparoscopic-assisted colorectal surgery. Lessons learned from 240 consecutive patients. Dis Colon Rectum 39: 155-159.
20. Monson JR, Hill AD, Darzi A (1995) Laparoscopic colonic surgery. Br J Surg 82: 150-157.
21. Ortega AE, Beart RW, Jr., Steele GD, Jr., Winchester DP, Greene FL (1995) Laparoscopic Bowel Surgery Registry. Preliminary results. Dis Colon Rectum 38: 681-686.
22. Pfeifer J, Wexner SD, Reissman P, et al. (1995) Laparoscopic vs open colon surgery. Costs and outcome. Surg Endosc 9: 1322-1326.
23. Phillips EH, Franklin M, Carroll BJ, et al. (1992) Laparoscopic colectomy. Ann Surg 216: 703-707.
24. Ramos JM, Beart RW, Jr., Goes R, Ortega AE, Schlinkert RT (1995) Role of laparoscopy in colorectal surgery. A prospective evaluation of 200 cases. Dis Colon Rectum 38: 494-501.
25. Reissman P, Cohen S, Weiss EG, Wexner SD (1996) Laparoscopic colorectal surgery: ascending the learning curve. World J Surg 20: 277-282.
26. Schlachta CM, Mamazza J, Poulin EC (1999) Laparoscopic sigmoid resection for acute and chronic diverticulitis. An outcomes comparison with laparoscopic resection for nondiverticular disease. Surg Endosc 13: 649-653.
27. Sher ME, Agachan F, Bortul M, et al. (1997) Laparoscopic surgery for diverticulitis. Surg Endosc 11: 264-267.
28. Smadja C, Sbai Idrissi M, Tahrat M, et al. (1999) Elective laparoscopic sigmoid colectomy for diverticulitis. Results of a prospective study. Surg Endosc 13: 645-648.
29. Tate JJ, Kwok S, Dawson JW, Lau WY, Li AK (1993) Prospective comparison of laparoscopic and conventional anterior resection. Br J Surg 80: 1396-1398.
30. Wexner SD, Reissman P, Pfeifer J, Bernstein M, Geron N (1996) Laparoscopic colorectal surgery: analysis of 140 cases. Surg Endosc 10: 133-136.

31. Schmitt SL, Cohen SM, Wexner SD, Nogueras JJ, Jagelman DG (1994) Does laparoscopic-assisted ileal pouch anal anastomosis reduce the length of hospitalization? Int J Colorectal Dis 9: 134-137.
32. Tucker JG, Ambroze WL, Orangio GR, et al. (1995) Laparoscopically assisted bowel surgery. Analysis of 114 cases. Surg Endosc 9: 297-300.
33. Schwandner O, Schiedeck TH, Bruch H (1999) The role of conversion in laparoscopic colorectal surgery: Do predictive factors exist? Surg Endosc 13: 151-156.
34. Slim K, Pezet D, Riff Y, Clark E, Chipponi J (1995) High morbidity rate after converted laparoscopic colorectal surgery. Br J Surg 82: 1406-1408.
35. Köckerling F, Schneider C, Reymond MA, et al. (1999) Laparoscopic resection of sigmoid diverticulitis. Results of a multicenter study. Laparoscopic Colorectal Surgery Study Group. Surg Endosc 13: 567-571.
36. Eypasch E, Tschubar F, Schmitz H, et al. (1999) Die minimalinvasive Therapie lohnt. Führen & Wirtschaft 1: 36.

Closing remarks and perspectives

Authors:

B. MILLAT, Surgical Unit, Hôpital St Eloi, Montpellier (France) ;

A. FINGERHUT, Surgical Unit, Centre Hospitalier Intercommunal de Poissy-St Germain, Poissy (France) ;

E. NEUGEBAUER, Biochemical and Experimental Division, 2nd Department of Surgery, University of Cologne (Germany) ;

Introduction

Obviously, the rationale for creating practice guidelines is to improve the quality of care we deliver to our patients. The efforts produced to ensure that the delivery of care takes into account the relevant evidence are praiseworthy. All EAES members will undoubtedly be grateful to those who participated in this systematic review of the literature, leading to recommendations explicitly linked to the supporting evidence. The success of such an endeavour was far from guaranteed at the beginning. The obstinacy of the organizing committee to drive the laparoscopic revolution, then bursting with innovation, and enthusiastic in the name of feasibility only, into the rigorous and potentially contentious requirements of evaluation has to be highlighted. Given the existence of diverse influences, laparoscopic surgery has been regarded by some of the medical community as a sort of perversion from traditional healthcare outcomes. From the depths of such disturbing accusations, this booklet is a brilliant response to its detractors. It is fairly certain that if it were not the burst of interest cast by the laparoscopic approach to so-called "common" operations such as appendectomy, inguinal hernia repair, or cholecystectomy, none of these tremendous efforts for evaluation would have been undertaken. Cause or consequence, laparoscopic surgery has undoubtedly been associated with irreversible changes in the overall management of modern surgical care. Even the most critical appraisal of this evolution cannot prevent recognizing that, at the very least, a large majority of these changes have fulfilled patients' expectancies.

How to produce guidelines?

"Most of the guidelines produced by specialty societies do not meet the basic principles of guideline development". This strong warning from Roberto Grilli and colleagues [1] could also be the conclusion from the critical appraisal of the consensus methods included in the present booklet. Bias is the chief enemy of science. The principal, identified shortcomings of the EAES consensus process are: biased panel selection, biased literature research [2], and lack of transparency in recommendations. Criticism is easy, while art is difficult ! Although the validity of the postal survey itself becomes questionable due to its low 14% response rate (see chapter 3), we have to take these criticisms into consideration for future improvement of the method. The key principles underpinning the development of guidelines are the multidisciplinarity of the panel, a quality-appraised systematic review of all the relevant published literature, and establishment of confidence levels [3] for recommendations based on the data analyzed. Each of these laudable aims would require additional comments that are beyond the scope of these conclusions. Just as an example, "multidisciplinarity" means implicating in the development of guidelines all the stakeholders who implement the recommendations, a much greater task

than just resolving the conflicts of interest inside the single-specialty group of EAES surgeons. A significant commitment of resources, manpower and time is required to complete guidelines. All those who feel concerned by the potential limitations in the impact of the present EAES guidelines should take an active part in the debate regarding the funding of the future development of the concept. Allocation of resources for the development of guidelines that meet quality requirements in order to lead to widespread ownership among the members of the association is the responsibility of the EAES administrative board. Feedback allowing assessment of the external validity of the guidelines will be the responsibility of each EAES member.

Do we need guidelines?

A surgeon is an artisan not an artist. The prerogative of an artist is the freedom to create. The prerogative of an artisan is the autonomy to choose the best solution from the external evidence for a specific, sometimes unique, situation. One, strong, limitation for appropriation of guidelines might stem from the misunderstanding of what they really are and what they should mean. Guidelines provide advice; they are not mandatory instructions. All those who try to produce guidelines from the best available external evidence are obviously conscious of the potential limitations associated with the applicability of conclusions derived from population studies to the unique, single, patient-doctor relationship. This recognition of the "Art" of medicine is explicit in the definition of evidence-based medicine itself: "the conscientious and judicious use of current best evidence from clinical care research in the management of individual patients." [4]. However, commentators [5] who express concern about the threat evidence-based medicine poses to the individual relationship doctors have with their patients, should think deeply and then express the same concern about the other threats to progress and clearly defined directions in the quality of care such as "eminence-based" medicine [3] and so-called "personal experience".

From the very beginning, medical practice has been learned through an apprenticeship process. Anecdotal cases, dogma, custom-based practice, clinical intuition and personal experience of the mentor were the "evidence" basis of teaching. The most striking observation derived from this approach is that it leads to a wide variability if not direct contradictions from one practice to another. Beliefs, intimate conviction and dogma constitute the "0" level of evidence.

When asked about their preferences among the different sources of evidence, 39% of responders indicate their "own experience" [6]. Although personal experience is of key importance to the technical aspects of surgery, one should accept with lucidity the weaknesses of our "personal experience" for evaluating the results of a specific procedure or the rationale for a specific indication. Even the small group of surgeons who accept the constraints of patient follow-up, do not always fulfil the validity requirements of recorded information: length and exhaustivity of follow-up, prospective collection of data, just to name two. Collection of all required data is one of the major pitfalls of the best clinical research trials. Rather than purporting their "experience" as a source of evidence, surgeons should, with due modesty, recognize that most of the time, if not always, they ignore their own results.

Failures of both "eminence-based" teaching and "personal experience" should be the main arguments for accepting the need of establishing objective guidelines for practice.

Another key point for accepting guidelines is the information explosion. Who can honestly pretend to be able to keep up with all the available sources of information ? It has been estimated that the mean reading time for the average clinical physician today is 30 minutes a week [7]. Groups such as the E.A.E.S. consensus conference have to collect and digest this information in order to produce evidence-based management guidelines. Obviously, bias in selection and analysis are difficult to eradicate. Even the most suspicious reader of guidelines has to recognize, however, that the relevance and validity of information that stem from this kind of critical appraisal of the literature might be more pertinent than "evidence" derived from original articles or traditional reviews.

Is the concept of consensus guidelines relevant for an European association?

The force behind the creation of guidelines is to decrease practice variations and slow the rising rate of health-care costs. Little information is availible as regards geographic variations of practice in Europe but it is easy to imagine that these variations do exist and that it seems unlikely that they can be explained only by variance in the incidence of disease. Moreover, strong differences may appear according to differences in surgeons' fields of competence, accreditation for practice, and last but not least, according to the differences in social health-care and reimbursement systems. Due to the growing importance of cost-effectiveness in surgical outcome evaluation, particularly in laparoscopic procedures, one should accept the potential limitations of guidelines when they refer explicitly to *one* specific health-care organization, as they might not be pertinent in some other healthcare system. The tremendous variations reported in hospital-stay or sick-leave duration for the same laparoscopic procedure among different European countries, for instance [8], strongly support this observation. Evaluating the relevance and validity of evidence based guidelines relative to the different European social systems could be a major contribution of our association for the future of Europe.

Where to go? The future development of the E.A.E.S. concept

The successful introduction of clinical guidelines is dependant on many factors including the clinical context and the methods of develoiping, disseminating, and implementing those guidelines [9]. The final most important question is whether a successful clinical practice guideline (CPG) development strategy and implemention influences clinical practice and improves outcome for patients. This question is yet unanswered, as such effects are difficult to prove.

Clinical decision-making is a combination of the patient's clinical and life situation, his or her preferences, evidence, health care setting, cultural values, and many other specific circumstances [7]. Through systematic and explicit methods, we can provide and organize information about the best care as suggested by scientific evidence [10].

The E.A.E.S. CDC concept has been critically evaluated at the 1999 annual meeting of the E.A.E.S. (see chapters 2 and 3). As a results it was concluded that changes in the methodological development and dissemination strategies are mandatory. Related to methodology, more rigorous methodological standards should be follwoed to ensure both the scientific quality and consensus quality in the development and revision of CPGs [11]. The quality of the consensus can be ensured through participation of all relevant stakeholders in the guideline panel and the application of formal consensus development methods. As the methodology is directly related to the impact of the guideline, it can be assumed that this type of "evidence-based consensus guidelines" possesses the highest level of scientific and political legitimacy.

However, it is not enough to concentrate only on methodology; the same energy must be put into dissemination and implementation. As thoroughly evaluated by Eypasch et al. [12] passive dissemination of information is generally ineffective. He could show that the actual impact of the CDC on reflux disease is negligible, even though in those who participated in the CDC. This, however, holds true also for other CDCs or guidelines developed outside the E.A.E.S.. Improved strategies have to be developed as already outlined by Grimshaw and Russell [13]. The executive committee of the E.A.E.S. decided to meet these new challenges – members of our Society are asked to support this endeavour in order to improve the care of our patients.

References

1. Grilli R, Magrini N, Penna A, Mura G, Liberati A (2000) Practice guidelines developed by specialty societies: the need for a critical appraisal. Lancet 355: 103-106.
2. Sauerland S, Neugebauer E (2000) Consensus conferences must include a systematic search and categorization of the evidence. Surg Endosc: (in press).
3. Fabian TC (1999) Evidence-based medicine in trauma care: whither goest thou? J Trauma 47: 225-232.

4. Davidoff F, Haynes B, Sackett D, Smith R (1995) Evidence based medicine. BMJ 310: 1085-1086.
5. McCormick J (1996) Death of the personal doctor. Lancet 348: 667-668.
6. Millat B, Fingerhut A, Flamant Y, et al. (1999) Survey of the impact of randomised clinical trials on surgical practice in France. Eur J Surg 165: 87-94.
7. Sackett DL, Richardson WS, Rosenberg W, Haynes RB, Evidence-based medicine: How to practice and teach EBM, Churchill Livingstone, London/UK, 1997
8. Fingerhut A, Millat B, Borrie F (1999) Laparoscopic versus open appendectomy: time to decide. World J Surg 23: 835-845.
9. Russell IT, Grimshaw JM, The effectiveness of referral guidelines: a review of methods and findings of published evaluations. In: Roland M, Coulter A (Eds.), Hospital referrals, Oxford University Press, Oxford/U.K., 1992, pp. 179-211.
10. Brouwers MC, Browman GP (1999) Development of clinical practice guidelines: surgical perspective. World J Surg 23: 1236-1241.
11. Helou A, Lorenz W, Ollenschläger G, Reinauer H, Schwartz FW (2000) Methodische Standards der Entwicklung evidenz-basierter Leitlinien in Deutschland. Konsens zwischen Wissenschaft, Selbstverwaltung und Praxis. Z Ärztl Fortbild Qualitätssich 94: 330-339.
12. Eypasch E, Thiel B, Sauerland S (2000) Laparoscopic fundoplication for gastro-oesophageal reflux disease – a consensus development conference and the evidence-based benefit. Langenbeck's Arch Surg 385: 57-63.
13. Grimshaw JM, Russell IT (1994) Achieving health gain through clinical guidelines. II: Ensuring guidelines change medical practice. Qual Health Care 3: 45-52.

Composition, photogravure et impression
JOUVE, 18, rue Saint-Denis, 75001 PARIS
N° 281492E — Dépot légal : Juin 2000